H. H. Allen

Allen's Compendium of Hardee's Tactics

Elementary instruction in the schools of the soldier, company and battalion

H. H. Allen

Allen's Compendium of Hardee's Tactics
Elementary instruction in the schools of the soldier, company and battalion

ISBN/EAN: 9783337309398

Printed in Europe, USA, Canada, Australia, Japan

Cover: Foto ©Paul-Georg Meister /pixelio.de

More available books at **www.hansebooks.com**

ALLEN'S COMPENDIUM

OF

HARDEE'S TACTICS.

ELEMENTARY INSTRUCTION

IN THE

SCHOOLS

OF THE

Soldier, Company and Battalion

WITH MANUAL OF ARMS

COMPILED BY H. H. ALLEN.

NEW YORK:
M. DOOLADY,
49 WALKER STREET.

1861.

TITLE FIRST.

Article First.

Formation of a Regiment in order of battle or in line.

1. A Regiment is composed of ten companies, which will habitually be posted from right to left, in the following order: first, sixth, fourth, ninth, third, eighth, fifth, tenth, seventh, second, according to the rank of captains.

2. With a less number of companies the same principle will be observed, viz.: the first captain will command the right company, the second captain the left company, the third captain the right centre company, and so on.

3. The companies thus posted will be designated from right to left, *first* company, *second* company, &c. This designation will be observed in the manœuvres.

4. The first two companies on the right, whatever their denomination, will form the *first division;* the next two companies the *second division;* and so on, to the left.

5. Each company will be divided into two equal parts, which will be designated as the first and second platoon, counting from the right; and each platoon, in like manner, will be subdivided into two sections.

6. In all exercises and manœuvres, every regiment, or part of a regiment, composed of two or more companies, will be designated as a battalion.

7. The color, with a guard to be hereinafter designated, will be posted on the left of the right centre battalion company. That company, and all on its right, will be denominated the *right wing* of the battalion; the remaining companies the *left wing*.

8. The formation of a regiment is in two ranks; and each company will be formed into two ranks, in the following manner: the corporals will be posted in the front rank, and on the right and left of platoons, according to height; the tallest corporal and the tallest man will form the first file, the next two tallest men will form the second file, and so on to the last file, which will be composed of the shortest corporal and the shortest man.

9. The odd and even files, numbered as one, two, in the company, from right to left, will form groups of four men, who will be designated *comrades in battle.*

10. The distance from one rank to another will be thirteen inches, measured from the breasts of the rear rank men to the backs or knapsacks of the front rank men.

11. For manœuvring, the companies of a battalion will always be equalized by transferring men from the strongest to the weakest companies.

Posts of Company Officers, Sergeants, and Corporals.

12. The company officers and sergeants are nine in number, and will be posted in the following manner:

13. The *captain* on the right of the company, touching with the left elbow.

14. The *first sergeant* in the rear rank, touching with the left elbow, and covering the captain. In the manœuvres he will be denominated *covering sergeant*, or *right guide* of the company.

15. The remaining officers and sergeants will be posted as file closers, and two paces behind the rear rank.

16. The *first lieutenant*, opposite the centre of the fourth section.

17. The *second lieutenant* opposite the centre of the first platoon.

18. The *third lieutenant*, opposite the centre of the second platoon.

19. The *second sergeant*, opposite the second file from the left of the company. In the manœuvres he will be designated *left guide* of the company.

20. The *third sergeant*, opposite the second file from the right of the second platoon.

21. The *fourth sergeant*, opposite the second file from the left of the first platoon.

22. The *fifth sergeant*, opposite the second file from the right of the first platoon.

23. In the left or tenth company of the battalion, the second sergeant will be posted in the front rank, and on the left of the battalion.

24. The corporals will be posted in the front rank, as prescribed No. 8.

25. Absent officers and sergeants will be replaced—officers by sergeants, and sergeants by corporals. The colonel may detach a first lieutenant from one company to command another, of which both the captain and first lieutenant are absent; but this authority will give no right to a lieutenant to demand to be so detached.

Article Second.

Instruction of the Battalion.

26. Every commanding officer is responsible for the instruction of his command. He will assemble the officers together for theoretical and practical instruction as often as he may judge necessary, and when unable to attend to this duty in person, it will be discharged by the officer next in rank.

27. Captains will be held responsible for the theoretical and practical instruction of their non-commissioned officers, and the adjutant for the instruction of the non-commissioned staff. To this end, they will require these tactics to be studied and recited lesson by lesson; and when instruction is given on the ground, each non-com-

missioned officer, as he explains a movement, should be required to put it into practical operation.

28. The non-commissioned officers should also be practised in giving commands. Each command, in a lesson, at the theoretical instruction, should first be given by the instructor, and then repeated, in succession by the non-commissioned officers, so that while they become habituated to the commands, uniformity may be established in the manner of giving them.

29. In the school of the soldier, the company officers will be the instructors of the squads; but if there be not a sufficient number of company officers present, intelligent sergeants may be substituted; and two or three squads, under sergeant instructors, be superintended, at the same time, by an officer.

30. Individual instruction being the basis of the instruction of companies, on which that of the regiment depends, and the first principles having the greatest influence upon this individual instruction, classes of recruits should be watched with the greatest care.

31. Instructors will explain, in a few clear and precise words, the movement to be executed; and, not to overburden the memory of the men, they will always use the same terms to explain the same principles.

32. They should often join example to precept, should keep up the attention of the men by an animated tone, and pass rapidly from one movement to another, as soon as that which they command has been executed in a satisfactory manner.

Instruction of Officers.

33. The instruction of officers can be perfected only by joining theory to practice. The Instructor will often practice them in marching and in estimating distances, and he will carefully endeavor to cause them to take steps equal in length and swiftness. They will also be exercised in the double quick step.

34. The instruction of officers will include all the Titles in this system of drill, and such regulations as prescribe their duties in peace and war.

Instruction of Sergeants.

35. As the discipline and efficiency of a company materially depend on the conduct and character of its sergeants, they should be selected with care, and properly instructed in all the duties appertaining to their rank.

Commands.

There are three kinds.

36. The command of *caution*, which is *attention.*

37. The *preparatory command*, which indicates the movement which is to be executed.

38. The command of *execution*, such as *march* or *halt*, or, in the manual of arms, the part of command which causes an execution.

39. The tone of command should be animated, distinct, and of a loudness proportioned to the number of men under instruction.

40. The command *attention* is pronounced at the top of the voice, dwelling on the last syllable.

41. The command of *execution* will be pronounced in a tone firm and brief.

42. The commands of caution and the preparatory commands are herein distinguished by *italics*, those of execution by CAPITALS.

43. Those preparatory commands which, from their length, are difficult to be pronounced at once, must be divided into two or three parts, with an ascending progression in the tone of command, but always in such a manner that the tone of execution may be more energetic and elevated; the divisions are indicated by a hyphen. The parts of commands which are placed in a parenthesis, are not pronounced.

TITLE SECOND.

SCHOOL OF THE SOLDIER.

General Rules and division of the School of the Soldier.

44. The object of this school being the individual and progressive instruction of the recruits, the instructor never requires a movement to be executed until he has given an exact explanation of it; and he executes, himself, the movement which he commands, so as to join example to precept. He accustoms the recruit to take, by himself, the position which is explained—teaches him to rectify it only when required by his want of intelligence—and sees that all the movements are performed without precipitation.

45. Each movement should be understood before passing to another. After they have been properly executed in the order laid down in each lesson, the instructor no longer confines himself to that order; on the contrary, he should change it, that he may judge of the intelligence of the men.

46. The instructor allows the men to rest at the end of each part of the lessons, and oftener, if he thinks proper, especially at the commencement; for this purpose he commands REST.

47. At the command REST, the soldier is no longer required to preserve immobility, or to remain in his place. If the instructor wishes merely to relieve the attention of the recruit, he commands, *in place*—REST; the soldier is then not required to preserve his immobility, but he always keeps one of his feet in its place.

48. When the instructor wishes to commence the instruction he commands—ATTENTION; at this command the soldier takes his position, remains motionless, and fixes his attention.

49. The *School of the Soldier* will be divided into three parts, the first, comprehending what ought to be taught to recruits without arms; the second, the manual of arms, the loadings and firings; the third, the principles of alignment, the march by the front, the different steps, the march by the flank, the principles of wheeling, and those of change

of direction; also, long marches in double quick time and the run.

50. Each part will be divided into lessons, as follows:

PART FIRST.

Lesson 1. Position of the soldier without arms: Eyes right, left and front.

Lesson 2. Facings.

Lesson 3. Principles of the direct step in common and quick time.

Lesson 4. Principles of the direct step in double quick time and the run.

PART SECOND.

Lesson 1. Principles of shouldered arms.

Lesson 2. Manual of arms.

Lesson 3. To load in four times, and at will.

Lesson 4. Firings, direct, oblique, by file, and by rank.

Lesson 5. To fire and load, kneeling and lying.

Lesson 6. Bayonet exercise.

PART THIRD.

Lesson 1. Union of eight or twelve men for instruction in the principles of alignment.

Lesson 2. The direct march, the oblique march, and the different steps.

Lesson 3. The march by the flank.

Lesson 4. Principles of wheeling and change of direction.

Lesson 5. Long marches in double quick time, and the run with arms and knapsacks.

PART FIRST.

51. This will be taught, if practicable, to one recruit at a time; but three or four may be united, when the number be great, compared with that of the instructors. In this case, the recruits will be placed in a single rank, at one pace from each other. In this part, the recruits will be without arms.

Lesson I.

Position of the Soldier.

52. Heels on the same line, as near each other as the conformation of the man will permit;

The feet turned out equally, and forming with each other something less than a right angle;

The knees straight without stiffness;

The body erect on the hips, inclining a little forward;

The shoulders square and falling equally;

The arms hanging naturally;

The elbows near the body;

The palm of the hand turned a little to the front, the little finger behind the seam of the pantaloons;

The head erect and square to the front, without constraint;

The chin near the stock, without covering it;

The eyes fixed straight to the front, and striking the ground about the distance of fifteen paces.

Remarks on the position of the Soldier.

Heels on the same line;

53. Because, if one were in the rear of the other, the shoulder on that side would be thrown back, or the position of the soldier would be constrained.

Heels more or less closed;

Because, men who are knock-kneed, or who

have legs with large calves, can not, without constraint, make their heels touch while standing.

The feet equally turned out, and not forming too large an angle;

Because, if one foot were turned out more than the other, a shoulder would be deranged, and if both feet be too much turned out, it would not be practicable to incline the upper part of the body forward, without rendering the whole position unsteady.

Knees extended without stiffness.

Because, if stiffened, constraint and fatigue would be unavoidable.

The body erect on the hips;

Because it gives equilibrium to the position. The instructor will observe that many recruits have the bad habit of dropping a shoulder, of drawing in a side, or of advancing a hip, particularly the right, when under arms. These are defects he will labor to correct.

The upper part of the body inclining forward.

Because, commonly, recruits are disposed to do the reverse, to project the belly, and to throw back the shoulders, when they wish to hold themselves erect, from which result great inconveniences in marching. The habit of inclining forward the upper part of the body is so important to contract, that the instructor must enforce it at the beginning, particularly with recruits who have naturally the opposite habit.

Shoulders square;

Because, if the shoulders be advanced beyond the line of the breast, and the back arched (the defect called *round-shouldered*, not uncommon among recruits), the man cannot align himself, nor use his piece with address. It is important, then, to correct this defect, and necessary to that end that the coat should sit easy about the shoulders and arm-pits; but in correcting this defect, the instructor will take care that the shoulders be not thrown too much to the rear, which would cause the belly to project, and the small of the back to be curved.

The arms hanging naturally, elbows near the body, the palm of the hand a little turned to the front, the little finger behind the seam of the pantaloons.

Because, these positions are equally important to the *shoulder-arms*, and to prevent the man from occupying more space in a rank than is necessary to the free use of the piece; they have, moreover, the advantage of keeping in the shoulders.

The face straight to the front, and without constraint;

Because, if there be stiffness in the latter position, it would communicate itself to the whole of the upper part of the body, embarrass its movements, and give pain and fatigue.

Eyes direct to the front;

Because, this is the surest means of maintaining the shoulders in line—an essential object, to be insisted on and attained.

54. The instructor having given the recruit the position of the soldier without arms, will

now teach him the turning of the head and eyes. He will command:

1. *Eyes*—Right. 2. Front.

55. At the word *right*, the recruit will turn the head gently, so as to bring the inner corner of the left eye in a line with the buttons of the coat, the eyes fixed on the line of the eyes of the men in, or supposed to be in, the same rank.

56. At the second command, the head will resume the direct or habitual position.

57. The movement of *Eyes*—Left will be executed by inverse means.

58. The instructor will take particular care that the movement of the head does not derange the squareness of the shoulders, which will happen if the movement of the former be too sudden.

59. When the instructor shall wish the recruit to pass from the state of attention to that of ease he will command:

Rest.

60. To cause a resumption of the habitual position, the instructor will command:

1. *Attention.* 2. SQUAD.

61. At the first word, the recruit will fix his attention; at the second, he will resume the prescribed position and steadiness.

LESSON II.

Facings.

62. Facings to the right and left will be executed in one *time*, or pause. The instructor will command:

1. *Squad.* 2. *Right* (or *left*)—FACE.

63. At the second command, raise the right foot slightly, turn on the left heel, raising the toes a little, and then replace the right heel by the side of the left, and on the same line.

64. The full face to the rear (or front) will be executed in two *times*, or pauses. The instructor will command:

1. *Squad.* 2. ABOUT—FACE.

65. (*First time.*) At the word *about*, the recruit will turn on the left heel, bring the left to the front, carry the right foot to the

rear, the hollow opposite to, and full three inches from, the left heel, the feet square to each other.

66. (*Second time*). At the word *face*, the recruit will turn on both heels, raise the toes a little, extend the hams, face to the rear, bringing, at the same time, the right heel by the side of the left.

67. The instructor will take care that these motions do not derange the position of the body.

Lesson III.

Principles of the Direct Step.

68. The length of the direct step, or pace, in common time, will be twenty-eight inches, reckoning from heel to heel, and in swiftness, at the rate of ninety in a minute.

69. The instructor, seeing the recruit confirmed in his position, will explain to him the principle and mechanism of this step—placing himself six or seven paces from, and facing to, the recruit. He will himself execute slowly the step in the way of illustration, and then command:

1. *Squad, forward.* 2. *Common time.*
3. MARCH.

70. At the first command, the recruit will throw the weight of the body on the right leg, without bending the left knee.

71. At the third command, he will smartly, but without a jerk, carry straight forward the left foot twenty-eight inches from the right, the sole near the ground, the ham extended, the toe a little depressed, and, as also the knee, slightly turned out; he will, at the same time, throw the weight of the body forward, and plant flat the left foot, without shock, precisely at the distance where it finds itself from the right when the weight of the body is brought forward, the whole of which will now rest on the advanced foot. The recruit will next, in like manner, advance the right foot and plant it as above, the heel twenty-eight inches from the heel of the left foot, and thus continue to march without crossing the legs, or striking the one against the other, without turning the shoulders, and preserving always the face direct to the front.

72. When the instructor shall wish to arrest the march, he will command:

1. *Squad.* 2. HALT.

73. At the second command, which will be given at the instant when either foot is coming to the ground, the foot in the rear will be brought up, and planted by the side of the other, without shock.

74. The instructor will indicate, from time to time, to the recruit, the cadence of the step by giving the command *one* at the instant of raising a foot, and *two* at the instant it ought to be planted, observing the cadence of ninety steps in a minute. This method will contribute greatly to impress upon the mind the two motions into which the step is naturally divided.

75. Common time will be employed only in the first and second parts of the School of the Soldier. As soon as the recruit has acquired steadiness, has become established in the principles of shouldered arms, and in the mechanism, length, and swiftness of the step in common time, he will be practised only in

quick time, the double quick time, and the run.

76. The principles of the step in quick time are the same as for common time, but its swiftness is at the rate of one hundred and ten steps per minute.

77. The instructor wishing the squad to march in quick time, will command:

1. *Squad, forward.* 2. MARCH.

LESSON IV.

Principles of the Double Quick Step.

78. The length of the double quick step is thirty-three inches, and its swiftness at the rate of one hundred and sixty-five steps per minute.

79. The instructor, wishing to teach the recruits the principles and mechanism of the double quick step, will command:

1. *Double Quick Step.* 2. MARCH.

80. At the first command, the recruit will raise his hands to a level with his hips, the hands closed, the nails towards the body, the elbows to the rear.

81. At the second command, he will raise to the front his left leg, bent, in order to give to the knee the greatest elevation, the part of the leg between the knee and the instep vertical, the toe depressed; he will then replace his foot in its former position; with the right leg he will execute what has just been prescribed for the left, and the alternate movement of the legs will be continued until the command:

1. *Squad.* 2. HALT.

82. At the second command, the recruit will bring the foot which is raised by the side of the other, and dropping at the same time his hands by his side, will resume the position of the soldier without arms.

83. The instructor, placing himself seven or eight paces from, and facing the recruit, will indicate the cadence by the commands *one* and *two*, given alternately, at the instant each foot should be brought to the ground, which at first will be in common time, but its rapidity will be gradually augmented.

84. The recruits being sufficiently estab-

lished in the principles of this step, the instructor will command:

1. *Squad, forward.* 2. *Double Quick.*
3. MARCH.

85. At the first command the recruit will throw the weight of his body on the right leg.

86. At the second command, he will place his arms as indicated in No. 80.

87. At the third command, he will carry forward the left foot, the leg slightly bent, the knee somewhat raised—will plant his left foot, the toe first, thirty-three inches from the right, and with the right foot will then execute what has just been prescribed for the left. This alternate movement of the legs will take place by throwing the weight of the body on the foot that is planted, and by allowing a natural, oscillatory motion to the arms.

88. The double quick step may be executed with different degrees of swiftness. Under urgent circumstances the cadence of this step may be increased to one hundred and eighty per minute. At this rate a distance of four

thousand yards would be passed over in about twenty-five minutes.

89. The recruits will be exercised also in running.

90. The principles are the same as for the double quick step, the only difference consisting in a greater degree of swiftness.

91. It is recommended, in marching at double quick time, or the run, that the men should breathe as much as possible through the nose, keeping the mouth closed. Experience has proved, that by conforming to this principle, a man can pass over a much longer distance, and with less fatigue.

PART SECOND.

To Mark Time.

92. The four men marching in the direct step, the instructor will command:

1. *Mark time.* 2. MARCH.

93. At the second command, which will be given at the instant a foot is coming to the

ground, the recruits will make a semblance of marching, by bringing the heels by the side of each other, and observing the cadence of the step, by raising each foot alternately without advancing.

94. The instructor wishing the direct step to be resumed, will command:

1. *Forward.* 2. MARCH.

95. At the second command, which will be given as prescribed above, the recruits will retake the step of twenty-eight inches.

To change step.

96. The squad being in march, the instructor will command:

1. *Change step.* 2. MARCH.

97. At the second command, which will be given at the instant either foot is coming to the ground, bring the foot which is in rear by the side of that which is in front, and step off again which was in front.

To march backwards.

98. The instructor wishing the squad to march backwards, will command:

1. *Squad backward.* 2. MARCH.

99. At the second command, the recruits will step off smartly with the left foot fourteen inches to the rear, reckoning from heel to heel, and so on with the feet in succession till the command *halt*, which will always be preceded by the caution *squad*. The men will halt at this command, and bring back the foot in front by the side of the other.

100. This step will always be executed in quick time.

101. The instructor will be watchful that the recruits march straight to the rear, and that the erect position of the body and the piece be not deranged.

PART THIRD.

102. When the recruits are well established in the *principles and mechanism of the step*, *the position of the body*, and *the manual of*

arms, the instructor will unite eight men, at least, and twelve men, at most, in order to teach them the principles of alignment, the principles of the touch of elbows in marching to the front, the principles of the march by the flank, wheeling from a halt, wheeling in marching, and the change of direction to the side of the guide. He will place the squad in one rank, elbow to elbow, and number the men from right to left.

Lesson I.

Alignments.

103. The instructor will at first teach the recruits to align themselves man by man, in order the better to make them comprehend the principles of alignment; to this end, he will command the two men on the right flank to march two paces to the front, and having aligned them, he will caution the remainder of the squad to move up, as they may be successively called, each by his number, and align themselves successively on the line of the first two men.

104. Each recruit, as designated by his number, will turn the head and eyes to the

right, as prescribed in the first lesson of the first part, and will march in *quick time two paces forward*, shortening the last, so as to find himself about six inches behind the new alignment, which he ought never to pass: he will next move up steadily by steps of two or three inches, the hams extending to the side of the man next to him on the alignment, so that, without deranging the head, the line of the eyes, or that of the shoulders, he may find himself in the exact line of his neighbor, whose elbow he will lightly touch without opening his own.

105. The instructor, seeing the rank well aligned, will command:

FRONT.

106. At this, the recruits will turn eyes to the front, and remain firm.

107. Alignments to the left will be executed on the same principles.

108. When the recruits shall have thus learned to align themselves, man by man, correctly, and without grouping or jostling, the instructor will cause the entire rank to align itself at once by the command:

Right (*or left*)—Dress.

109. At this, the rank, except the two men placed in advance as a basis of alignment, will move up in *quick time*, and place themselves on the new line, according to the principles prescribed in No. 78.

110. The instructor, placed five or six paces in front, and facing the rank, will carefully observe that the principles are followed, and then pass to the flank that has served as the basis, to verify the alignment.

111. The instructor, seeing the greater number of the rank aligned, will command:

Front.

112. The instructor may afterwards order *this* or *that* file *forward* or *back*, designating each by its number. The file or files designated, only, will slightly turn the head towards the basis, to judge how much they ought to move up or back, steadily place themselves on the line, and then turn eyes to the front, without a particular command to that effect.

113. Alignments to the rear will be execu-

ted on the same principles, the recruits stepping back a little beyond the line, and then dressing up according to the principles prescribed No. 3, the instructor commanding:

Right (*or left*) *backward*—DRESS.

114. After each alignment, the instructor will examine the position of the men, and cause the rank to come to *ordered arms*, to prevent too much fatigue, and also the danger of negligence at *shouldered arms*.

LESSON II.

115. The men having learned, in the first and second parts, to march with steadiness in common time, and to take steps equal in length and swiftness, will be exercised in the third part only in *quick time*, *double quick time*, and the *run*; the instructor will cause them to execute successively, at these different gaits, the march to the front, the facing about in marching, the march by the flank, the wheels at a halt and in marching, and the changes of direction to the side of the guide.

116. The instructor will inform the recruits

that at the command *march*, they will always move off in *quick time*, unless this command should be preceded by that of *double quick*.

To march to the front.

117. The rank being correctly aligned, when the instructor shall wish to cause it to march by the front, he will place a well instructed man on the right or the left, according to the side on which he may wish the guide to be, and command:

1. *Squad, forward.* 2. *Guide right* (or *left*).
3. MARCH.

118. At the command *march*, the rank will step off smartly with the left foot; the guide will take care to march straight to the front, keeping his shoulders always in a square with that line.

119. The instructor will observe, in marching to the front, that the men touch lightly the elbow towards the side of the guide; that they do not open out the left elbow, nor the right arm; that they yield to pressure coming from the side of the guide, and resist that coming from the opposite side; that they re-

cover, by insensible degrees, the slight touch of the elbow, if lost; that they maintain the head direct to the front, no matter on which side the guide may be; and if found before or behind the alignment, that the man in fault corrects himself by shortening or lengthening the step, by degrees almost insensible.

120. The instructor will labor to cause recruits to comprehend that the alignment can only be preserved, in marching, by the regularity of the step, the touch of the elbow, and the maintenance of the shoulders in a square with the line of direction; that if, for instance, the step of some be longer than that of others, or if some march faster than others, a separation of elbows, and the loss of the alignment, would be inevitable; that if (it being required that the head should be direct to the front) they do not strictly observe the touch of elbows, it would be impossible for an individual to judge whether he marches abreast with his neighbor or not, and whether there be not an interval between them.

121. The impulsion of the quick step having a tendency to make men too easy and free in their movements, the instructor will be careful

to regulate the cadence of this step, and to habituate them to preserve always the erectness of the body, and the due length of the pace.

122. The men being well established in the principles of the direct march, the instructor will exercise them in marching obliquely. The rank being in march, the instructor will command:

1. *Right* (or *left*) *oblique*. 2. MARCH.

123. At the second command, each man will make a half face to the right (or left), and will then march straight forward in the new direction. As the men no longer touch elbows, they will glance along the shoulders of the nearest files, towards the side to which they are obliquing, and will regulate their steps so that the shoulders shall always be behind that of their next neighbor on that side, and that his head shall conceal the heads of the other men in the rank. Besides this, the men should preserve the same length of pace, and the same degree of obliquity.

124. The instructor, wishing to resume the primitive direction, will command:

1. *Forward.* 2. MARCH.

125. At the second command, each man will make a half face to the left (or right), and all will then march straight to the front, conforming to the principles of the direct march.

To march to the front in double quick time.

126. When the several principles, heretofore explained, have become familiar to the recruits, and they shall be well established in the position of the body, the bearing of arms, and the mechanism, length, and swiftness of the step, the instructor will pass them from *quick* to *double quick* time, and the reverse, observing not to make them march obliquely in double quick time, till they are well established in the cadence of this step.

127. The squad being at a march in quick time, the instructor will command:

1. *Double quick.* 2. MARCH.

128. At the command *march*, which will be given when either foot is coming to the ground, the squad will step off in double quick time. The men will endeavor to follow the

principles laid down in the first part of this book, and to preserve the alignment.

129. When the instructor wishes the squad to resume the step in quick time, he will command:

1. *Quick time.* 2. MARCH.

130. At the command *march*, which will be given when either foot is coming to the ground, the squad will retake the step in quick time.

131. The squad being in march, the instructor will halt it by the commands and means prescribed Nos. 72 and 73. The command *halt* will be given an instant before the foot is ready to be placed on the ground.

132. The squad being in march in double quick time, the instructor will occasionally cause it to mark time by the commands prescribed No. 92. The men will then mark double quick time, without altering the cadence of the step. He will also cause them to pass from the direct to the oblique step, and reciprocally, conforming to what has been prescribed No. 123, and following.

133. The squad being at a halt, the in-

structor will cause it to march in double quick time, by preceding the command *march*, by *double quick*.

134. The instructor will endeavor to regulate well the cadence of this step.

To face about in marching.

135. If the squad be marching in quick, or double quick time, and the instructor should wish to march it in retreat, he will command:

1. *Squad right about.* 2. MARCH.

136. At the command *march*, which will be given at the instant the left foot is coming to the ground, the recruit will bring this foot to the ground, and turning on it, will face to the rear; he will then place the right foot in the new direction, and step off with the left foot.

To march backwards.

137. The squad being at a halt, if the instructor should wish to march it in the back step, he will command:

1. *Squad backward.* 2. *Guide left* (or *right.*) 3. MARCH.

138. The back step will be executed by the means prescribed No. 98.

139. The instructor, in this step, will be watchful that the men do not lean on each other.

140. As the march to the front in quick time should only be executed at shouldered arms, the instructor, in order not to fatigue the men too much, and also to prevent negligence in gait and position, will halt the squad from time to time, and cause arms to be ordered.

141. In marching at *double quick time*, the men will always carry their pieces on the *right shoulder*, or at a *trail. This rule is general.*

142. If the instructor shall wish the pieces carried at a trail, he will give the command *trail arms*, before the command *double quick.* If, on the contrary, this command be not given, the men will shift their pieces to the right shoulder at the command *double quick.* In either case, at the command *halt*, the men

will bring their pieces to the position of *shoulder arms. This rule is general.*

Lesson III.

The march by flank.

143. The rank being at a halt, and correctly aligned, the instructor will command:

1. *Squad, right*—Face. 2. *Forward.*
3. March.

144. At the last part of the first command, the rank will face to the right; the even numbered men, after facing to the right, will step quickly to the right side of the odd numbered men, the latter standing fast, so that when the movement is executed, the men will be formed into files of two men abreast.

145. At the third command, the squad will step off smartly with the left foot; the files keeping aligned, and preserving their intervals.

146. The march by the left flank will be executed by the same commands, substituting the word *left* for *right*, and by inverse

means; in this case, the even numbered men, after facing to the left, will stand fast, and the odd numbered will place themselves on their left.

147. The instructor will place a well-instructed soldier by the side of the recruit who is at the head of the rank, to regulate the step, and to conduct him; and it will be enjoined on this recruit to march always elbow to elbow with the soldier.

148. The instructor will cause to be observed in the march, by the flank, the following rules:

That the step be executed according to the principles prescribed for the direct step:

Because these principles, without which men, placed elbow to elbow, in the same rank, cannot preserve unity and harmony of movement, are of a more necessary observance in marching in file.

That the head of the man who immediately precedes, covers the heads of all who are in front:

Because it is the more certain rule by which each man may maintain himself in the exact line of the file.

149. The instructor will place himself habitually five or six paces on the flank of the rank marching in file, to watch over the execution of the principles prescribed above. He will also place himself sometimes in its rear, halt, and suffer it to pass fifteen or twenty paces, the better to see whether the men cover each other accurately.

150. When he shall wish to halt the rank, marching by the flank, and to cause it to face to the front, he will command:

1. *Squad.* 2. HALT. 3. FRONT.

151. At the second command, the rank will halt, and afterwards no man will stir, although he may have lost his distance. This prohibition is necessary, to habituate the men to a constant preservation of their distances.

152. At the third command, each man will front by facing to the left, if marching by the right flank, and by a face to the right, if marching by the left flank. The rear rank men will at the same time move quickly into their places, so as to form the squad again into one rank.

153. When the men have become accustomed to marching by the flank, the instructor will cause them to change direction by file; for this purpose, he will command:

1. *By file left* (or *right.*) 2. MARCH.

154. At the command *march*, the first file will change direction to the left (or right), in describing a small arc of a circle, and will then march straight forward; the two men of this file, in wheeling, will keep up the touch of the elbows, and the man on the side to which the wheel is made, will shorten the first three or four steps. Each file will come successively to wheel on the same spot where that which preceded it wheeled.

The instructor will also cause the squad to face by the right or left flank, in marching, and for this purpose will command:

1. *Squad by the right* (or *left*) *flank.*
2. MARCH.

155. At the second command, which will be given a little before either foot comes to the ground, the recruits will turn the body,

plant the foot that is raised in the new direction, and step off with the other foot without altering the cadence of the step; the men will double or undouble rapidly.

156. If, in facing by the right or the left flank, the squad should face to the rear, the men will come into one rank, agreeably to the principles indicated No. 152. It is to be remarked that it is the men who are in rear who always move up to form into single rank, and in such manner as never to invert the order of the numbers in the rank.

157. If, when the squad has been faced to the rear, the instructor should cause it to face by the left flank, it is the even numbers who will double by moving to the left of the odd numbers; but if by the right flank, it is the odd numbers who will double to the right of the even numbers.

158. This lesson, like the preceding one, will be practiced with pieces at the shoulder; but the instructor may, to give relief by change, occasionally order *support arms*, and he will require of the recruits marching in this position, as much regularity as in the former.

The march by the flank in double quick time.

159. The principles of the march by the flank, in double quick time, are the same as in quick time. The instructor will give the commands prescribed No. 351, taking care always to give the command *double quick* before that of *march.*

160. He will pay the greatest attention to the cadence of the step.

161. The instructor will cause the change of direction, and the march by the flank, to be executed in double quick time, by the same commands, and according to the same principles as in quick time.

162. The instructor will cause the pieces to be carried either on the *right-shoulder*, or at a *trail.*

163. The instructor will sometimes march the squad by the flank, without doubling the files.

164. The principles of this march are the same as in two ranks, and it will always be executed in quick time.

165. The instructor will give the commands prescribed No. 155, but he will be careful to caution the squad not to double files.

166. The instructor will be watchful that the men do not bend their knees unequally, which would cause them to tread on the heels of the men in front, and also to lose the cadence of the step and their distances.

167. The various movements in this lesson will be executed in single rank. In the changes of direction, the leading man will change direction without altering the length or the cadence of the step. The instructor will recall to the attention of the men, that in facing by the right or left flank, in marching, they will not double, but march in one rank.

Lesson IV.

WHEELINGS.

General principles of Wheeling.

168. Wheelings are of two kinds; from halts, or on fixed pivots, and in march, or on movable pivots.

169. Wheeling on a fixed pivot takes place in passing a corps from the order in battle to the order in column, or from the latter to the former.

170. Wheels in marching take place in changes of direction in column, as often as this movement is executed to the side opposite to the guide.

171. In wheels from a halt, the pivot-man only turns in his place, without advancing or receding.

172. In the wheels in marching, the pivot takes steps of nine or eleven inches, according as the squad is marching in quick or double-quick time, so as to clear the wheeling-point, which is necessary, in order that the sub-divisions of a column may change direction without losing their distances, as will be explained in the School of the Company.

173. The man on the wheeling flank will take the full step of twenty-eight inches, or thirty-three inches, according to the gait.

Wheeling from a halt, or on a fixed pivot.

174. The rank being at a halt, the instructor will place a well-instructed man on the wheeling flank to conduct it, and then command:

1. *By squad, right wheel.* 2. MARCH.

175. At the second command, the rank will

step off with the left foot, turning at the same time the head a little to the left, the eyes fixed on the line of the eyes of the men to their left; the pivot-man will merely mark time in gradually turning his body, in order to conform himself to the movement of the marching flank; the man who conducts this flank will take steps of twenty-eight inches, and from the first step advance a little the left shoulder, cast his eyes from time to time along the rank, and feel constantly the elbow of the next man lightly, but never push him.

176. The other men will feel lightly the elbow of the next man towards the pivot, resist pressure coming from the opposite side, and each will conform himself to the marching flank—shortening his step according to his approximation to the pivot.

177. The instructor will make the rank wheel round the circle once or twice before halting, in order to cause the principles to be the better understood, and he will be watchful that the centre does not break.

178. He will cause the wheel to the left to be executed according to the same principles.

179. When the instructor shall wish to arrest the wheel, he will command:

1. *Squad.* 2. HALT.

180. At the second command, the rank will halt, and no man stir. The instructor, going to the flank opposite the pivot, will place the two outer men of that flank in the direction he may wish to give to the rank, without, however, displacing the pivot, who will conform the line of his shoulders to this direction. The instructor will take care to have between these two men and the pivot, only the space necessary to contain the other men. He will then command

Left (or *right*)—DRESS.

181. At this the rank will place itself on the alignment of the two men established as the basis, in conformity with the principles prescribed.

182. The instructor will next command FRONT, which will be executed as prescribed, No. 314.

Remarks on the principles of the wheel from a halt.

183. *Turn a little the head towards the marching*

flank, and fix the eyes on a line of the eyes of the men who are on that side.

Because, otherwise, it would be impossible for each man to regulate the length of his step so as to conform his own movement to that of the marching flank.

Touch lightly the elbow of the next man towards the pivot;

In order that the files may not open out in the wheel.

Resist pressure that comes from the side of the marching flank;

Because, if this principle be neglected, the pivot, which ought to be a fixed point, in wheels from a halt, might be pushed out of its place by pressure.

Wheeling in marching, or on a movable pivot.

184. When the recruits have been brought to execute well the wheel from a halt, they will be taught to wheel in marching.

185. To this end, the rank being in march, when the instructor shall wish to cause it to change direction to the reverse flank (to the

side opposite to the guide or pivot flank), he will command:

1. *Right* (or *left*) *wheel*. 2. MARCH.

186. The first command will be given when the rank is yet *four* paces from the wheeling point.

187. At the second command, the wheel will be executed in the same manner as from a halt, except that the touch of the elbow will remain towards the marching flank (or side of the guide), instead of the side of the actual pivot; that the pivot man, instead of merely turning in his place, will conform himself to the movement of the marching flank, feel lightly the elbow of the next man, take steps of full nine inches, and thus gain ground forward in describing a small curve so as to clear the point of the wheel. The middle of the rank will bend slightly to the rear. As soon as the movement shall commence, the man who conducts the marching flank will cast his eyes on the ground over which he will have to pass.

188. The wheel being ended, the instructor will command:

1. *Forward.* 2. March.

189. The first command will be pronounced when *four* paces are yet required to complete the change of direction.

190. At the command *march*, which will be given at the instant of completing the wheel, the man who conducts the marching flank will direct himself straight forward; the pivot man and all the rank will retake the step of twenty-eight inches, and bring the head direct to the front.

Turning, or change of direction to the side of the guide.

191. The change of direction to the side of the guide, in marching, will be executed as follows: The instructor will command:

1. *Left* (or *right*) *turn.* 2. March.

192. The first command will be given when the rank is yet *four* paces from the turning point.

193. At the command *march*, to be pronounced at the instant the rank ought to turn, the guide will face to the left (or right) in

marching, and move forward in the new direction without slackening or quickening the cadence, and without shortening or lengthening the step. The whole rank will promptly conform itself to the new direction; to effect which, each man will advance the shoulder opposite to the guide, take the double quick step, to carry himself in the new direction, turn the head and eyes to the side of the guide, and retake the touch of the elbow on that side, in placing himself on the alignment of the guide, from whom he will take the step, and then resume the direct position of the head. Each man will thus arrive successively on the alignment.

Wheeling and changing direction to the side of the guide, in double quick time.

194. When the recruits comprehend and execute well, in quick time, the wheels at a halt and in marching, and the change of direction to the side of the guide, the instructor will cause the same movements to be repeated in double quick time.

195. These various movements will be exe-

cuted by the same commands and according to the same principles as in quick time, except that the command *double quick* will precede that of *march*. In wheeling while marching, the pivot man will take steps of eleven inches, and in the changes of direction to the side of the guide, the men on the side opposite the guide must increase the gait in order to bring themselves into line.

MANUAL OF ARMS.

LESSON FIRST.

Principles of Shouldered Arms.

1. THE recruit being placed as explained in the first lesson of the first part, the instructor will cause him to bend the right arm slightly, and place the piece in it, in the following manner:

2. The piece in the right hand—the barrel nearly vertical, and resting in the hollow of the shoulder—the guard to the front, the arm hanging nearly at its full length near the body; the thumb and fore-finger embracing the guard, the remaining fingers closed together, and grasping the swell of the stock just under the cock, which rests on the little finger.

3. Recruits are frequently seen with natural defects in the conformation of the shoulders, breast, and hips. These the instructor will labor to correct in the lessons without

arms, and afterwards, by steady endeavors, so that the appearance of the pieces, in the same line, may be uniform, and this without constraint to the men in their positions.

4. The instructor will have occasion to remark that recruits, on first bearing arms, are liable to derange their position by lowering the right shoulder and the right hand, or by sinking the hip, and spreading out the elbows.

5. He will be careful to correct all these faults by continually rectifying the position; he will sometimes take away the piece to replace it the better; he will avoid fatiguing the recruits too much in the beginning, but labor by degrees to render this position so natural and easy that they may remain in it a long time without fatigue.

6. Finally, the instructor will take great care that the piece, at a shoulder, be nót carried too high nor too low: if too high, the right elbow would spread out, the soldier would occupy too much space in his rank, and the piece be made to waver; if too low, the files would be too much closed, the soldier would not have the necessary space to handle

his piece with facility, the right arm would become too much fatigued, and would draw down the shoulder.

7. The instructor, before passing to the second lesson, will cause to be repeated the movements of *eyes right*, *left*, and *front*, and the *facings*.

LESSON SECOND.

Manual of Arms.

8. The manual of arms will be taught to four men, placed, at first, in one rank, elbow to elbow, and afterwards in two ranks.

9. Each command will be executed in one *time* (or pause), but this time will be divided into motions, the better to make known the mechanism.

10. The rate (or swiftness) of each motion, in the manual of arms, with the exceptions herein indicated, is fixed at the ninetieth part of a minute; but, in order not to fatigue the attention, the instructor will, at first, look more particularly to the execution of the motions, without requiring a nice observance of

the cadence, to which he will bring the recruits progressively, and after they shall have become a little familiarized with the handling of the piece.

11. As the motions relative to the cartridge, to the rammer, and to the fixing and unfixing of the bayonet, cannot be executed at the rate prescribed, nor even with a uniform swiftness, they will not be subjected to that cadence. The instructor will, however, labor to cause these motions to be executed with promptness, and, above all, with regularity.

12. The last syllable of the command will decide the brisk execution of the first motion of each time (or pause). The commands *two*, *three*, and *four*, will decide the brisk execution of the other motions. As soon as the recruits shall well comprehend the positions of the several motions of a time, they will be taught to execute the time without resting on its different motions; the mechanism of the time will nevertheless be observed, as well to give a perfect use of the piece, as to avoid the sinking of, or slurring over, either of the motions.

13. The manual of arms will be taught in the following progression: The instructor will command:

Support—Arms.

One time and three motions.

14. (*First motion.*) Bring the piece, with the right hand, perpendicularly to the front and between the eyes, the barrel to the rear; seize the piece with the left hand at the lower band, raise this hand as high as the chin, and seize the piece at the same time with the right hand four inches below the cock.

15. (*Second motion.*) Turn the piece with the right hand, the barrel to the front; carry the piece to the left shoulder, and pass the fore-arm extended on the breast, between the right hand and the cock; support the cock against the left fore-arm, the left hand resting on the right breast.

16. (*Third motion.*) Drop the right hand by the side.

17. When the instructor may wish to give repose in this position, he will command:

Rest.

18. At this command the recruits will bring up smartly the right hand to the handle of the piece (small of the stock), when they will not be required to preserve silence, or steadiness of position.

19. When the instructor may wish the recruits to pass from this position to that of silence and steadiness, he will command:

1. *Attention.* 2. Squad.

20. At the second word, the recruits will resume the position of the third motion of *support arms.*

Shoulder—Arms.

One time and three motions.

21. (*First motion.*) Grasp the piece with the right hand under and against the left fore-arm; seize it with the left hand at the lower band, the thumb extended; detach the piece slightly from the shoulder, the left fore-arm along the stock.

22. (*Second motion.*) Carry the piece vertically to the right shoulder with both hands, the rammer to the front, change the position of the right hand so as to embrace the guard with the thumb and fore-finger, slip the left hand to the height of the shoulder, the fingers extended and joined, the right arm nearly straight.

23. (*Third motion.*) Drop the left hand quickly by the side.

Present—ARMS.

One time and two motions.

24. (*First motion.*) With the right hand bring the piece erect before the centre of the body, the rammer to the front; at the same time seize the piece with the left hand half way between the guide sight and lower band, the thumb extended along the barrel and against the stock, the fore-arm horizontal and resting against the body, the hand as high as the elbow.

25. (*Second motion.*) Grasp the small of the stock with the right hand below and against the guard.

Shoulder—Arms.

One time and two motions.

26. (*First motion.*) Bring the piece to the right shoulder, at the same time change the position of the right hand so as to embrace the guard with the thumb and forefinger, slip up the left hand to the height of the shoulder, the fingers extended and joined, the right arm nearly straight.

27. (*Second motion.*) Drop the left hand quickly by the side.

Order—Arms.

One time and two motions.

28. (*First motion.*) Seize the piece briskly with the left hand near the upper band, and detach it slightly from the shoulder with the right hand; loosen the grasp of the right hand, lower the piece with the left, re-seize the piece with the right hand above the lower band, the little finger in rear of the barrel, the butt about four inches from the ground,

the right hand supported against the hip, drop the left hand by the side.

29. (*Second motion.*) Let the piece slip through the right hand to the ground, by opening slightly the fingers, and take the position about to be described.

Position of order arms.

30. The hand low, the barrel between the thumb and fore-finger extended along the stock; the other fingers extended and joined; the muzzle about two inches from the right shoulder; the rammer in front; the toe (or beak) of the butt, against, and in a line with, the toe of the right foot, the barrel perpendicular.

31. When the instructor may wish to give repose in this position, he will command:

REST.

32. At this command, the recruits will not be required to preserve silence or steadiness.

33. When the instructor may wish the recruits to pass from this position to that of silence and steadiness, he will command:

1. *Attention.* 2. SQUAD.

34. At the second word, the recruits will resume the position of *order arms.*

Shoulder—ARMS.

One time and two motions.

35. (*First motion.*) Raise the piece vertically with the right hand to the height of the right breast, and opposite the shoulder, the elbow close to the body; seize the piece with the left hand below the right, and drop quickly the right hand to grasp the piece at the swell of the stock, the thumb and fore-finger embracing the guard; press the piece against the shoulder with the left hand, the right arm nearly straight.

36. (*Second motion.*) Drop the left hand quickly by the side.

Load in nine times.

1. LOAD.*

One time and one motion.

37. Grasp the piece with the left hand as high as the right elbow, and bring it vertically opposite the middle of the body, shift the right hand to the upper band, place the butt between the feet, the barrel to the front; seize it with the left hand near the muzzle, which should be three inches from the body; carry the right hand to the cartridge box.

2. *Handle*—CARTRIDGE.

One time and one motion.

38. Seize the cartridge with the thumb and next two fingers, and place it between the teeth.

3. *Tear*—CARTRIDGE.

One time and one motion.

39. Tear the paper to the powder, hold the

---

* Whenever the loadings and firings are to be executed, the instructor will cause the cartridge boxes to be brought to the front.

cartridge upright between the thumb and first two fingers, near the top; in this position place it in front of and near the muzzle —the back of the hand to the front.

4. *Charge*—CARTRIDGE.

One time and one motion.

40. Empty the powder into the barrel: disengage the ball from the paper with the right hand and the thumb and first two fingers of the left; insert it into the bore, the pointed end uppermost, and press it down with the right thumb; seize the head of the rammer with the thumb and fore-finger of the right hand, the other fingers closed, the elbows near the body.

5. *Draw*—RAMMER.

One time and three motions.

41. (*First motion.*) Half draw the rammer by extending the right arm; steady it in this position with the left thumb; grasp the rammer near the muzzle with the right hand,

the little finger uppermost, the nails to the front, the thumb extended along the rammer.

42. (*Second motion.*) Clear the rammer from the pipes by again extending the arm, the rammer in the prolongation of the pipes.

43. (*Third motion.*) Turn the rammer, the little end of the rammer passing near the left shoulder; place the head of the rammer on the ball, the back of the hand to the front.

6. *Ram*—CARTRIDGE.

One time and one motion.

44. Insert the rammer as far as the right, and steady it in this position with the thumb of the left hand; seize the rammer at the small end with the thumb and fore-finger of the right hand, the back of the hand to the front; press the ball home, the elbows near the body.

7. *Return*—RAMMER.

One time and three motions.

45. (*First motion.*) Draw the rammer half way out, and steady it in this position with

the left thumb; grasp it near the muzzle with the right hand, the little finger uppermost, the nails to the front, the thumb along the rammer; clear the rammer from the bore by extending the arm, the nails to the front, the rammer in the prolongation of the bore.

46. (*Second motion.*) Turn the rammer, the head of the rammer passing near the left shoulder, and insert it in the pipes until the right hand reaches the muzzle, the nails to the front.

47. (*Third motion.*) Force the rammer home by placing the little finger of the right hand on the head of the rammer; pass the left hand down the barrel to the extent of the arm, without depressing the shoulder.

8. Prime.*

One time and two motions.

48. (*First motion.*) With the left hand raise the piece till the hand is as high as the eye, grasp the small of the stock with the right hand; half face to the right; place, at

---

* If Maynard's primer be used, the command will be, *load in eight times*, and the eighth command will be,

the same time, the right foot behind and at right angles with the left; the hollow of the right foot against the left heel. Slip the left hand down to the lower band, the thumb along the stock, the left elbow against the body; bring the piece to the right side, the butt below the right fore-arm—the small of the stock against the body and two inches below the right breast, the barrel upwards, the muzzle on a level with the eye.

49. (*Second motion.*) Half cock with the thumb of the right hand, the fingers supported against the guard and the small of the stock—remove the old cap with one of the fingers of the right hand, and with the thumb and fore-finger of the same hand take a cap from the pouch, place it on the nipple, and press it down with the thumb; seize the small of the stock with the right hand.

---

shoulder arms, and executed from *return rammer*, in one time and two motions as follows:

(*First motion.*) Raise the piece with the left hand, and take the position of shoulder arms, as indicated No. 145.

(*Second motion.*) Drop the left hand quickly by the side.

9. *Shoulder*—Arms.

One time and two motions.

50. (*First motion.*) Bring the piece to the right shoulder and support it there with the left hand, face to the front; bring the right heel to the side of and on a line with the left; grasp the piece with the right hand as indicated in the position of *shoulder arms.*

51. (*Second motion.*) Drop the left hand quickly by the side.

Ready.

One time and three motions.

52. (*First motion.*) Raise the piece slightly with the right hand, making a half face to the right on the left heel; carry the right foot to the rear, and place it at right angles to the left, the hollow of it opposite to, and against the left heel; grasp the piece with the left hand at the lower band and detach it slightly from the shoulder.

53. (*Second motion.*) Bring down the piece with both hands, the barrel upwards, the left thumb extended along the stock, the butt below the right forearm, the small of the stock against the body, and two inches below the right breast, the muzzle as high as the eye, the left elbow against the side; place at the same time the right thumb on the head of the cock, the other fingers under and against the guard.

54. (*Third motion.*) Cock, and seize the piece at the small of the stock, without deranging the position of the butt.

Aim.

One Time and One Motion.

55. Raise the piece with both hands, and support the butt against the right shoulder; the left elbow down, the right as high as the shoulder; incline the head upon the butt, so that the right eye may perceive quickly the notch of the hausse, the front sight, and the object aimed at; the left eye closed, the right thumb extended along the stock, the fore-finger on the trigger.

56. When recruits are formed in two ranks, to execute the firings, the front rank men will raise a little less the right elbow, in order to facilitate the aim of the rear rank men.

57. The rear rank men, in aiming, will each carry the right foot about eight inches to the right, and towards the left heel of the man next on the right, inclining the upper part of the body forward.

Fire.

One time and one motion.

58. Press the fore-finger against the trigger, fire, without lowering or turning the head, and remain in this position.

59. Instructors will be careful to observe when the men fire, that they aim at some distinct object, and that the barrel be so directed that the line of fire and the line of sight be in the same vertical plane. They will often cause the firing to be executed on ground of different inclinations, in order to accustom the men to fire at objects either above or below them.

LOAD.

One time and one motion.

60. Bring down the piece with both hands, at the same time face to the front and take the position of *load*, as indicated No. 156. Each rear rank man will bring his right foot by the side of the left.

61. The men being in this position, the instructor will cause the loading to be continued by the commands and means prescribed No. 156 and following.

62. If, after firing, the instructor should not wish the recruits to reload, he will command:

Shoulder—ARMS.

One time and one motion.

63. Throw up the piece briskly with the left hand and resume the position of *shoulder arms*, at the same time face to the front, turning on the left heel, and bring the right heel on a line with the left.

64. To accustom the recruits to wait for the command *fire*, the instructor, when they are in the position of *aim*, will command:

Recover—ARMS.

One time and one motion.

65. At the first part of the command, withdraw the finger from the trigger; at the command *arms*, retake the position of the third motion of *ready*.

66. The recruits being in the position of the third motion of *ready*, if the instructor should wish to bring them to a shoulder, he will command:

Shoulder—ARMS.

One time and one motion.

67. At the command *shoulder*, place the thumb upon the cock, the fore-finger on the trigger, half-cock, and seize the small of the stock with the right hand. At the command *arms*, bring up the piece briskly to the right shoulder, and retake the position of shoulder arms.

68. The recruits being at shoulder arms, when the instructor shall wish to fix bayonets, he will command:

Fix—Bayonet.

One time and three motions.

69. (*First motion.*) Grasp the piece with the left hand at the height of the shoulder, and detach it slightly from the shoulder with the right hand.

70. (*Second motion.*) Quit the piece with the right hand, lower it with the left hand, opposite the middle of the body, and place the butt between the feet without shock; the rammer to the rear, the barrel vertical, the muzzle three inches from the body; seize it with the right hand at the upper band, and carry the left hand reversed to the handle of the sabre-bayonet.

71. (*Third motion.*) Draw the sabre-bayonet from the scabbard, and fix it on the extremity of the barrel; seize the piece with the left hand, the arm extended, the right hand at the upper band.

Shoulder—Arms.

One time and two motions.

72. (*First motion.*) Raise the piece with the left hand, and place it against the right shoulder, the rammer to the front; seize the piece at the same time with the right hand at the swell of the stock, the thumb and forefinger embracing the guard, the right arm nearly extended.

73. (*Second motion.*) Drop briskly the left hand by the side.

Charge—Bayonet.

One time and two motions.

74. (*First motion.*) Raise the piece slightly with the right hand, and make a half face to the right on the left heel; place the hollow of the right foot opposite to, and three inches from the left heel, the feet square; seize the piece at the same time with the left hand a little above the lower band.

75. (*Second motion.*) Bring down the piece with both hands, the barrel uppermost, the

left elbow against the body; seize the small of the stock, at the same time, with the right hand, which will be supported against the hip; the point of the sabre-bayonet as high as the eye.

Shoulder—ARMS.

One time and two motions.

76. (*First motion.*) Throw up the piece briskly with the left hand in facing to the front, place it against the right shoulder, the rammer to the front; turn the right hand so as to embrace the guard, slide the left hand to the height of the shoulder, the right hand nearly extended.

77. (*Second motion.*) Drop the left hand smartly by the side.

Trail—ARMS.

One time and two motions.

78. (*First motion.*) The same as the first motion of *order arms.*

79. (*Second motion.*) Incline the muzzle

slightly to the front, the butt to the rear, and about four inches from the ground. The right hand supported at the hip, will so hold the piece that the rear rank men may not touch with their bayonets the men in the front rank.

Shoulder—ARMS.

80. At the command *shoulder*, raise the piece perpendicularly in the right hand, the little finger in rear of the barrel; at the command *arms*, execute what has been prescribed for the *shoulder* from the position of *order arms*.

Unfix—BAYONET.

One time and three motions.

81. (*First and second motions.*) The same as the first and second motions of *fix bayonet*, except that, at the end of the second command, the thumb of the right hand will be placed on the spring of the sabre-bayonet, and the left hand will embrace the handle of the sabre-bayonet and the barrel, the thumb extended along the blade.

82. (*Third motion.*) Press the thumb of the right hand on the spring, wrest off the sabre-bayonet, turn it to the right, the edge to the front, lower the guard until it touches the right hand, which will seize the back and the edge of the blade between the thumb and first two fingers, the other fingers holding the piece; change the position of the hand without quitting the handle, return the sabre-bayonet to the scabbard, and seize the piece with the left hand, the arm extended.

Shoulder—Arms.

One time and two motions.

83. (*First motion.*) The same as the first motion from *fix bayonet*, No. 191.

84. (*Second motion.*) The same as the second motion from *fix bayonet*, No. 192.

Secure—Arms.

One time and three motions.

85. (*First motion.*) The same as the first motion of *support arms*, No. 133, except with the right hand seize the piece at the small of the stock.

86. (*Second motion.*) Turn the piece with both hands, the barrel to the front; bring it opposite the left shoulder, the butt against the hip, the left hand at the lower band, the thumb as high as the chin, and extended on the rammer; the piece erect and detached from the shoulder; the left fore-arm against the piece.

87. (*Third motion.*) Reverse the piece, pass it under the left arm, the left hand remaining at the lower band, the thumb on the rammer, to prevent it from sliding out; the little finger resting against the hip, the right hand falling at the same time by the side.

Shoulder—Arms.

One time and three motions

88. (*First motion.*) Raise the piece with the left hand, and seize it with the right hand at the small of the stock. The piece erect and detached from the shoulder, the butt against the hip, the left fore-arm along the piece.

89. (*Second motion.*) The same as the second motion of *shoulder arms from a support.*

90. (*Third motion.*) The same as the third motion of *shoulder arms from a support.*

Right shoulder shift—Arms.

One time and two motions.

91. (*First motion.*) Detach the piece perpendicularly from the shoulder with the right hand, and seize it with the left between the lower band and guide-sight, raise the piece, the left hand at the height of the shoulder and four inches from it; place, at the same time, the right hand on the butt, the beak between the first two fingers, the other two fingers under the butt plate.

92. (*Second motion.*) Quit the piece with the left hand, raise and place the piece on the right shoulder with the right hand, the lock plate upwards; let fall, at the same time, the left hand by the side.

Shoulder—ARMS.

One time and two motions.

93. (*First motion.*) Raise the piece perpendicularly by extending the right arm to its full length, the rammer to the front, at the same time seize the piece with the left hand between the lower band and guide sight.

94. (*Second motion.*) Quit the butt with the right hand, which will immediately embrace the guard, lower the piece to the position of shoulder arms, slide up the left hand to the height of the shoulder, the fingers extended and closed. Drop the left hand by the side.

95. The men being at support arms, the instructor will sometimes cause pieces to be brought to the right shoulder. To this effect, he will command:

Right shoulder shift—ARMS.

One time and two motions.

96. (*First motion.*) Seize the piece with the right hand, below and near the left fore-

arm, place the left hand under the butt, the heel of the butt between the first two fingers.

97. (*Second motion.*) Turn the piece with the left hand, the lock plate upwards, carry it to the right shoulder, the left hand still holding the butt, the muzzle elevated; hold the piece in this position, and place the right hand upon the butt, as is prescribed No. 210, and let fall the left hand by the side.

Support—Arms.

One time and two motions.

98. (*First motion.*) The same as the first motion of *shoulder arms*, No. 212.

99. (*Second motion.*) Turn the piece with both hands, the barrel to the front, carry it opposite the left shoulder, slip the right hand to the small of the stock, place the left fore-arm extended on the breast as is prescribed No. 134, and let fall the right hand by the side.

Arms—AT WILL.

One time and one motion.

100. At this command, carry the piece at pleasure on either shoulder, with one or both hands, the muzzle elevated.

Shoulder—ARMS.

One time and one motion.

101. At this command, retake quickly the position of shoulder arms.

102. The recruits being at ordered arms, when the instructor shall wish to cause the pieces to be placed on the ground, he will command:

Ground—ARMS.

One time and two motions.

103. (*First motion.*) Turn the piece with the right hand, the barrel to the left, at the same time seize the cartridge box with the left hand, bend the body, advance the left foot, the heel opposite the lower band; lay the piece on

the ground with the right hand, the toe of the butt on a line with the right toe, the knees slightly bent, the right heel raised.

104. (*Second motion.*) Rise up, bring the left foot by the side of the right, quit the cartridge box with the left hand, and drop the hands by the side.

Raise—Arms.

One time and two motions.

105. (*First motion.*) Seize the cartridge box with the left hand, bend the body, advance the left foot opposite the lower band, and seize the piece with the right hand.

106. (*Second motion.*) Raise the piece, bringing the left foot by the side of the right; turn the piece with the right hand, the rammer to the front; at the same time quit the cartridge box with the left hand, and drop this hand by the side.

Inspection of Arms.

107. The recruits being at *ordered arms*, and having the sabre-bayonet in the scab-

bard, if the instructor wishes to cause an inspection of arms, he will command:

Inspection—Arms.

One time and two motions.

108. (*First motion*) Seize the piece with the left hand below and near the upper band, carry it with both hands opposite the middle of the body, the butt between the feet, the rammer to the rear, the barrel vertical, the muzzle about three inches from the body; carry the left hand reversed, to the sabre-bayonet, draw it from the scabbard and fix it on the barrel; grasp the piece with the left hand below and near the upper band, seize the rammer with the thumb and fore-finger of the right hand bent, the other fingers closed.

109. (*Second motion.*) Draw the rammer as has been explained in *loading*, and let it glide to the bottom of the bore, replace the piece with the left hand opposite the right shoulder and retake the position of *ordered arms.*

110. The instructor will then inspect in succession the piece of each recruit, in pass-

ing along the front of the rank. Each, as the instructor reaches him, will raise smartly his piece with his right hand, seize it with the left between the lower band and guide sight, the lock to the front, the left hand at the height of the chin, the piece opposite to the left eye; the instructor will take it with the right hand at the handle, and, after inspecting it, will return it to the recruit, who will receive it back with the right hand, and replace it in the position of *ordered arms.*

111. When the instructor shall have passed him, each recruit will retake the position prescribed at the command *inspection arms*, return the rammer, and resume the position of *ordered arms.*

112. If, instead of *inspection of arms*, the instructor should merely wish to cause bayonets to be fixed, he will command:

Fix—BAYONET.

113. Take the position indicated No. 227, fix bayonets as has been explained, and immediately resume the position of *ordered arms.*

114. If it be the wish of the instructor, after firing, to ascertain whether the pieces have been discharged, he will command:

Spring—RAMMERS.

115. Put the rammer in the barrel as has been explained above, and immediately retake the position of *ordered arms.*

116. The instructor, for the purpose stated, can take the rammer by the small end, and spring it in the barrel, or cause each recruit to make it ring in the barrel.

117. Each recruit, after the instructor passes him, will return rammer, and resume the position of *ordered arms.*

Remarks on the Manual of Arms.

118. The manual of arms frequently distorts the persons of recruits, before they acquire ease and confidence in the several positions. The instructor will therefore frequently recur to elementary principles in the course of the lessons.

119. Recruits are also extremely liable to

curve the sides and back, and to derange the shoulders, especially in loading. Consequently the instructor will not cause them to dwell too long at a time, in one position.

120. When, after some days of exercise in the manual of arms, the four men shall be well established in their use, the instructor will always terminate the lesson by marching the men for some time in one rank, and at one pace apart, in common and quick time, in order to confirm them more and more in the mechanism of the step; he will also teach them to mark time and to change step, which will be executed in the following manner:

To mark time.

121. The four men marching in the direct step, the instructor will command:

1. *Mark time.* 2. MARCH.

122. At the second command, which will be given at the instant a foot is coming to the ground, the recruits will make a semblance of marching, by bringing the heels by the side of

each other, and observing the cadence of the step, by raising each foot alternately without advancing.

123. The instructor wishing the direct step to be resumed, will command:

1. *Forward.* 2. MARCH.

124. At the second command, which will be given as prescribed above, the recruits will retake the step of twenty-eight inches.

To change step.

125. The squad being in march, the instructor will command:

1. *Change step.* 2. MARCH.

126. At the second command, which will be given at the instant either foot is coming to the ground, bring the foot which is in rear by the side of that which is in front, and step off again with the foot which was in front.

To march backwards.

127. The instructor wishing the squad to march backwards, will command:

1. *Squad backward.* 2. MARCH.

128. At the second command, the recruits will step off smartly with the left foot fourteen inches to the rear, reckoning from heel to heel, and so on with the feet in succession till the command *halt*, which will always be preceded by the caution *squad.* The men will halt at this command, and bring back the foot in front by the side of the other.

129. This step will always be executed in quick time.

130. The instructor will be watchful that the recruits march straight to the rear, and that the erect position of the body and the piece be not deranged.

LESSON THIRD.

To load in four times.

131. The object of this lesson is to prepare the recruits to load at will, and to cause them to distinguish the times which require the greatest regularity and attention, such as

charge cartridge, *ram cartridge*, and *prime*. It will be divided as follows:

132. The first time will be executed at the end of the command; the three others at the commands, *two*, *three*, and *four*.

The instructor will command:

1. *Load in four times.* 2. LOAD.

133. Execute the times to include charge cartridge.

TWO.

134. Execute the times to include ram cartridge.

THREE.

135. Execute the times to include prime.

FOUR.

136. Execute the time of *shoulder arms*.

To load at will.

137. The instructor will next teach loading at will, which will be executed as loading in four times, but continued, and without resting on either of the times. He will command:

1. *Load at will.* 2. LOAD.

138. The instructor will habituate the recruits, by degrees, to load with the greatest possible promptitude, each without regulating himself by his neighbor, and above all without waiting for him.

139. The cadence prescribed No. 129, is not applicable to loading in four times, or at will.

LESSON FOURTH.

Firings.

140. The firings are direct or oblique, and will be executed as follows:

The direct fire.

141. The instructor will give the following commands:

1. *Fire by Squad.* 2. *Squad.* 3. READY.
4. AIM. 5. FIRE. 6. LOAD.

142. These several commands will be exe-

cuted as has been prescribed in the *Manual of Arms.* At the third command the men will come to the position of *ready* as heretofore explained. At the fourth they will aim according to the rank in which each may find himself placed, the rear rank men inclining forward a little the upper part of the body, in order that their pieces may reach as much beyond the front rank as possible.

143. At the sixth command, they will load their pieces and return immediately to the position of *ready.*

144. The instructor will recommence the firing by the commands:

1. *Squad.* 2. Aim. 3. Fire. 4. Load.

145. When the instructor wishes the firing to cease, he will command:

Cease firing.

146. At this command the men will cease firing, but will load their pieces if unloaded, and afterwards bring them to a shoulder.

Oblique Firings.

147. The oblique firings will be executed to the right and left, and by the same commands as the direct fire, with this single difference—the command *aim* will always be preceded by the caution, *right* or *left oblique.*

Position of the two ranks in the Oblique Fire to the right.

148. At the command *ready*, the two ranks will execute what has been prescribed for the direct fire.

149. At the cautionary command, *right oblique*, the two ranks will throw back the right shoulder and look steadily at the object to be hit.

150. At the command *aim* each front rank man will aim to the right without deranging the feet; each rear rank man will advance the left foot about eight inches towards the right heel of the man next on the right of his file leader and aim to the right, inclining the upper part of the body forward and bending a little the left knee.

Position of the two ranks in the Oblique Fire to the left.

151. At the cautionary command *left oblique*, the two ranks will throw back the left shoulder and look steadily at the object to be hit.

152. At the command *aim*, the front rank will take aim to the left, without deranging the feet; each man in the rear rank will advance the right foot about eight inches towards the right heel of the man next on the right of his file leader, and aim to the left, inclining the upper part of the body forward and bending a little the right knee.

153. In both cases, at the command *load*, the men of each rank will come to the position of load as prescribed in the direct fire; the rear rank men bringing back the foot which is to the right and front by the side of the other. Each man will continue to load as if isolated.

To fire by file.

154. The fire by file will be executed by the two ranks, the files of which will fire suc-

cessively, and without regulating on each other, except for the first fire.

155. The instructor will command:

1. *Fire by file.* 2. *Squad.* 3. *Ready.*
4. COMMENCE FIRING.

156. At the third command, the two ranks will take the position prescribed in the direct fire.

157. At the fourth command, the file on the right will aim and fire; the rear rank man, in aiming, will take the position indicated No. 176.

158. The men of this file will load their pieces briskly, and fire a second time; reload, and fire again, and so on in continuation.

159. The second file will aim at the instant the first brings down pieces to reload, and will conform in all respects to that which has just been prescribed for the first file.

160. After the first fire, the front and rear rank men will not be required to fire at the same time.

161. Each man, after loading, will return to the position of ready, and continue the fire.

162. When the instructor wishes the fire to cease, he will command:

Cease—FIRING.

163. At this command, the men will cease firing. If they have fired, they will load their pieces, and bring them to a shoulder; if at the position of *ready*, they will half-cock and shoulder arms; if in the position of *aim*, they will bring down their pieces, half-cock, and shoulder arms.

To fire by rank.

164. The fire by rank will be executed by each entire rank alternately.

165. The instructor will command:

1. *Fire by rank.* 2. *Squad.* 3. READY. 4. *Rear rank.* 5. AIM. 6. FIRE. 7. LOAD.

166. At the third command, the two ranks will take the position of *ready*, as prescribed in the direct fire.

167. At the seventh command, the rear rank will execute that which has been prescribed in the direct fire, and afterwards take the position of *ready*.

168. As soon as the instructor sees several men of the rear rank in the position of ready, he will command:

1. *Front Rank.* 2. AIM. 3. FIRE.
4. LOAD.

169. At these commands, the men in the front rank will execute what has been prescribed for the rear rank, but they will not step off with the right foot.

170. The instructor will recommence the firing by the rear rank, and will thus continue to alternate from rank to rank, until he shall wish the firing to cease, when he will command, *cease firing*, which will be executed as heretofore prescribed.

LESSON FIFTH.

To fire and load kneeling.

171. In this exercise the squad will be supposed loaded and drawn up in one rank. The instruction will be given to each man individually, without times or motions, and in the following manner:

172. The instructor will command:

FIRE AND LOAD KNEELING.

173. At this command, the man on the right of the squad will move forward three paces, and halt; then carry the right foot to the rear and to the right of the left heel, and in a position convenient for placing the right knee upon the ground in bending the left leg; place the right knee upon the ground; lower the piece, the left fore-arm supported upon the thigh on the same side, the right hand on the small of the stock, the butt resting on the right thigh, the left hand supporting the piece near the lower band.

174. He will next move the right leg to the left around the knee supported on the ground, until this leg is nearly perpendicular to the direction of the left foot, and thus seat himself comfortably on the right heel.

175. Raise the piece with the right hand and support it with the left, holding it near the lower band, the left elbow resting on the left thigh, near the knee; seize the hammer with the thumb, the forefinger under the guard, cock and seize the piece at the small of the stock; bring the piece to the shoulder, *aim* and *fire.*

176. Bring the piece down as soon as it is fired, and support it with the left hand, the butt resting against the right thigh; carry the piece to the rear, rising on the knee, the barrel downwards, the butt resting on the ground, in this position support the piece with the left hand, at the upper band, draw cartridge with the right and load the piece, ramming the ball, if necessary, with both hands.

177. When loaded, bring the piece to the front with the left hand, which holds it at the upper band; seize it at the same time with

the right hand at the small of the stock; turn the piece, the barrel uppermost and nearly horizontal, the left elbow resting on the left thigh; half-cock, remove the old cap and prime, rise, and return to the ranks.

178. The second man will then be taught what has just been prescribed for the first, and so on through the remainder of the squad.

To fire and load lying.

179. In this exercise the squad will be in one rank and loaded; the instruction will be given individually and without times or motions.

180. The instructor will command:

FIRE AND LOAD LYING.

181. At this command, the man on the right of the squad will move forward three paces and halt; he will then bring his piece to an order, drop on both knees, and place himself on the ground, flat on his belly. In this position he will support the piece nearly horizontal with the left hand, holding it near

the lower band, the butt end of the piece and the left elbow resting on the ground, the barrel uppermost, cock the piece with the right hand, and carry this hand to the small of the stock; raise the piece with both hands, press the butt against the shoulder, and resting on both elbows, *aim* and *fire*.

182. As soon as he has fired, bring the piece down, and turn upon his left side, still resting on his left elbow; bring back the piece until the cock is opposite his breast, the butt end resting on the ground; take out a cartridge with the right hand; seize the small of the stock with this hand, holding the cartridge with the thumb and first two fingers; he will then throw himself on his back, still holding the piece with both hands; carry the piece to the rear, place the butt between the heels, barrel up, the muzzle elevated. In this position, charge cartridge, draw rammer, ram cartridge, and return rammer.

183. When finished loading, the man will turn again upon his left side, remove the old cap and prime, then raise the piece vertically,

rise, turn about, and resume his position in the ranks.

184. The second man will be taught what has just been prescribed for the first, and so on throughout the squad.

LESSON SIXTH.

Bayonet Exercise.

185. The bayonet exercise in this book will be confined to two movements, the *guard against infantry*, and the *guard against cavalry.* The men will be placed in one rank, with two paces interval, and being at shoulder arms, the instructor will command:

1. *Guard against Infantry.* 2. GUARD.

One time and two motions.

186. (*First motion.*) Make a half face to the right, turning on both heels, the feet square to each other; at the same time raise the piece slightly, and seize it with the left hand above and near the lower band.

187. (*Second motion.*) Carry the right foot twenty inches perpendicularly to the rear, the right heel on the prolongation of the left, the knees slightly bent, the weight of the body resting equally on both legs; lower the piece with both hands, the barrel uppermost, the left elbow against the body; seize the piece at the same time with the right hand at the small of the stock, the arms falling naturally, the point of the bayonet slightly elevated.

Shoulder—ARMS.

One time and one motion.

188. Throw up the piece with the left hand, and place it against the right shoulder, at the same time bring the right heel by the side of the left and face to the front.

1. *Guard against Cavalry.* 2. GUARD.

One time and two motions.

189. Both motions the same as for *guard against infantry*, except that the right hand will be supported against the hip, and the

bayonet held at the height of the eye, as in *charge bayonet.*

Shoulder—Arms.

One time and one motion.

190. Spring up the piece with the left hand, and place it against the right shoulder, at the same time bring the right heel by the side of the left, and face to the front.

SCHOOL OF THE COMPANY.

General Rules and division of the School of the Company.

1. Instruction by company shall always precede that of battalion, and the object being to prepare the soldiers for the higher school, the exercises of detail by company will be strictly adhered to, as well in respect to principles, as the order of progression herein prescribed.

2. There will be attached to a company undergoing elementary instruction, a captain, a covering sergeant, and a certain number of file closers, the whole posted in the manner indicated: Title first, and, according to the same Title, the officer charged with the exercise of such company will herein be denominated the *instructor*.

3. The company will always be formed in two ranks. The instructor will then cause the files to be numbered, and for this purpose will command:

In each rank—Count Twos.

4. At this command, the men count in each rank, from right to left, pronouncing in a loud and distinct voice, in the same tone, without hurry and without turning the head, *one*, *two*, according to the place which each one occupies. He will also cause the company to be divided into platoons and sections, taking care that the first platoon is always composed of an even number of files.

5. The instructor will be as clear and concise as possible in his explanations; he will cause faults of detail to be rectified by the captain, to whom he will indicate them, if the captain should not have himself observed them; and the instructor will not otherwise interfere, unless the captain should not well comprehend, or should badly execute his intentions.

6. Composure, or presence of mind, in him who commands, and in those who obey, being the first means of order in a body of troops, the instructor will labor to habituate the company in this essential quality, and will himself give the example.

LESSON FIRST.

Article First.

To open ranks.

7. The company being at ordered arms, the ranks and file closers well aligned, when the instructor shall wish to cause the ranks to be opened, he will direct the left guide to place himself on the left of the front rank, which being executed, he will command:

1. *Attention.* 2. *Company.* 3. *To the rear.* 4. *Open order.*

8. At the fourth command, the covering sergeant and the left guide will step off smartly to the rear, four paces from the front rank, in order to mark the alignment of the rear rank. They will judge this distance by the eye, without counting the steps.

9. The instructor will place himself at the same time on the right flank, in order to observe, if these two non-commissioned officers are on a line parallel to the front rank, and if necessary, to correct their positions, which being executed, he will command:

5. MARCH.

10. At this command, the front rank will stand fast.

11. The rear rank will step to the rear, without counting their steps, and will place themselves on the alignment marked for this rank, conforming to what is prescribed in the School of the Soldier, No. 99.

12. The covering sergeant will align the rear rank on the left guide placed to mark the left of this rank.

13. The file closers will march to the rear at the same time with the rear rank, and will place themselves two paces from this rank when it is aligned.

14. The instructor seeing the rear rank aligned, will command:

6. FRONT.

15. At this command, the sergeant on the left of the rear rank will return to his place as a file closer.

16. The rear rank being aligned, the instructor will direct the captain and the covering sergeant to observe the men in their re-

spective ranks, and to correct, if necessary, the positions of persons and pieces.

LESSON SECOND.

Article First.

To advance in line of battle.

17. The company being in line of battle, and correctly aligned, when the instructor shall wish to exercise it in marching by the front, he will assure himself that the shoulders of the captain and covering sergeant are perfectly in the direction of their respective ranks, and that the sergeant accurately covers the captain; the instructor will then place himself twenty-five or thirty paces in front of them, face to the rear, and place himself exactly on the prolongation of the line passing between their heels.

18. The instructor, being aligned on the directing file, will command:

1. *Company, forward.*

19. At this, a sergeant, previously designated, will move six paces in advance of the

captain: the instructor, from the position prescribed, will correctly align this sergeant on the prolongation of the directing file.

20. This advanced sergeant, who is to be charged with the direction, will, the moment his position is assured, take two points on the ground in the straight line which would pass between his own and the heels of the instructor.

21. These dispositions being made, the instructor will step aside and command.

2. March.

22. At this, the company will step off with life. The directing sergeant will observe, with the greatest precision, the length and cadence of the step, marching on the two points he has chosen; he will take in succession, and always a little before arriving at the point nearest to him, new points in advance, exactly in the same line with the first two, and at the distance of some fifteen or twenty paces from each other. The captain will march steadily in the trace of the directing sergeant, keeping always six paces from him; the men will each maintain the head direct to the front, feel lightly the elbow of his

neighbor on the side of direction, and conform himself to the principles prescribed, School of the Soldier, for the march by the front.

23. The man next to the captain will take special care not to pass him; to this end, he will keep the line of his shoulders a little in the rear, but in the same direction with those of the captain.

24. The file closers will march at the habitual distance of two paces behind the rear rank.

25. If the men lose the step, the instructor will command:

To the—STEP.

26. At this command, the men will glance towards the directing sergeant, retake the step from him, and again direct their eyes to the front.

27. The instructor will cause the captain and covering sergeant to be posted sometimes on the right, and sometimes on the left of the company.

28. The directing sergeant, in advance, having the greatest influence on the march of the company, he will be selected for the pre-

cision of his step, his habit of maintaining his shoulders in a square with a given line of direction, and of prolonging that line without variation.

29. If this sergeant should fail to observe these principles, undulations in the front of the company must necessarily follow; the men will be unable to contract the habit of taking steps equal in length and swiftness, and of maintaining their shoulders in a square with the line of direction—the only means of attaining perfection in the march in line.

30. The instructor, with a view the better to establish the men in the length and cadence of the step, and in the principles of the march in line, will cause the company to advance three or four hundred paces, at once, without halting, if the ground will permit. In the first exercises he will march the company with open ranks, the better to observe the two ranks.

31. The instructor will see, with care, that all the principles of the march in line are strictly observed; he will generally be on the directing flank, in a position to observe the two ranks, and the faults they may commit;

he will sometimes halt behind the directing file during some thirty successive steps, in order to judge whether the directing sergeant, or the directing file, deviate from the perpendicular.

Article Second.

To halt the company marching in line of battle, and to align it.

32. The instructor, wishing to halt the company, will command:

1. *Company.* 2. Halt.

33. At the second command, the company will halt; the directing sergeant will remain in advance, unless ordered to return to the line of file closers. The company being at a halt, the instructor may advance the first three or four files on the side of direction, and align the company on that basis, or he may confine himself to causing the alignment to be rectified. In this last case, he will command: *Captain, rectify the alignment.* The captain will direct the covering sergeant to attend to the rear rank, when each, glancing his eyes along his rank, will promptly rectify it, conforming

to what is prescribed in the School of the Soldier, No. 193.

Article Third.

Oblique march in line of battle.

34. The company being in the direct march, when the instructor shall wish to cause it to march obliquely, he will command:

1. *Right* (or *left*) *oblique.* 2. March.

35. At the command *march*, the company will take the oblique step. The men will accurately observe the principles prescribed in the School of the Soldier, No. 123. The rear rank men will preserve their distances, and march in rear of the man next on the right (or left) of their habitual file leaders.

36. When the instructor wishes the direct march to be resumed, he will command:

1. *Forward.* 2. March.

37. At the command *march*, the company will resume the direct march. The instructor will move briskly twenty paces in front of the captain, and facing the company, will place himself exactly in the prolongation of the cap-

tain and covering sergeant; and then, by a sign, will move the directing sergeant on the same line, if he be not already on it; the latter will immediately take two points on the ground between himself and the instructor, and as he advances, will take new points of direction, as is explained No. 53.

38. In the oblique march, the men not having the touch of elbows, the guide will always be on the side towards which the oblique is made, without any indication to that effect being given; and when the direct march is resumed, the guide will be, equally without indication, on the side where it was previous to the oblique.

39. The instructor will, at first, cause the oblique to be made towards the side of the guide. He will also direct the captain to have an eye on the directing sergeant, in order to keep on the same perpendicular line to the front with him, while following a parallel direction.

40. During the continuance of the march, the instructor will be watchful that the men follow parallel directions, in conforming to the principles prescribed in the School of the

Soldier, for preserving the general alignment; whenever the men lose the alignment, he will be careful that they regain it by lengthening or shortening the step, without altering the cadence, or changing the direction.

41. The instructor will place himself in front of the company, and face to it, in order to regulate the march of the directing sergeant, or the man who is on the flank towards which the oblique is made, and to see that the principles of the march are properly observed, and that the files do not crowd.

Article Fourth.

To mark time, to march in double quick time, and the back step.

42. The company being in the direct march, and in quick time, the instructor, to cause it to mark time, will command:

1. *Mark time.* 2. March.

43. To resume the march, he will command:

1. *Forward.* 2. March.

44. To cause the march in double quick time, the instructor will command:

1. *Double quick.* 2. MARCH.

45. The command *march* will be pronounced at the instant either foot is coming to the ground.

46. To resume quick time, the instructor will command:

1. *Quick time.* 2. MARCH.

47. The command *march* will be pronounced at the instant either foot is coming to the ground.

48. The company being at a halt, the instructor may cause it to march in the back step; to this effect, he will command:

1. *Company backward.* 2. MARCH.

49. The back step will be executed according to the principles prescribed in the School of the Soldier, No. 99, but the use of it being rare, the instructor will not cause more than fifteen or twenty steps to be taken in succession, and to that extent but seldom.

50. The instructor ought not to exercise the company in marching in double quick time till the men are well established in the length and swiftness of the pace in quick time: he will then endeavor to render the march of

one hundred and sixty-five steps in the minute equally easy and familiar, and also cause them to observe the same erectness of body and composure of mind, as if marching in quick time.

51. When marching in double quick time, if a subdivision (in a column) has to change direction by *turning*, or has to form into line, the men will quicken the pace to one hundred and eighty steps in a minute. The same swiftness of step will be observed under all circumstances where great rapidity of movement is required. But as ranks of men can not march any length of time at so swift a rate, without breaking or confusion, this acceleration will not be considered a prescribed exercise, and accordingly companies or battalions will only be habitually exercised in the double quick time of one hundred and sixty-five steps in the minute.

Article Fifth.

To march in retreat.

52. The company being halted and correctly aligned, when the instructor shall wish to cause it to march in retreat, he will command:

1. *Company.* 2. *About*—FACE.

53. The company having faced to the rear, the instructor will place himself in front of the directing file, conforming to what is prescribed, No. 136.

54. The instructor, being correctly established on the prolongation of the directing file, will command:

3. *Company, forward.*

55. At this, the directing sergeant will conform himself to what is prescribed, No. 56, with this difference—he will place himself six paces in front of the line of file closers, now leading.

56. The covering sergeant will step into the line of file closers, opposite to his interval, and the captain will place himself in the rear rank, now become the front.

57. This disposition being promptly made, the instructor will command:

4. MARCH.

58. At this, the directing sergeant, the captain, and the men, will conform themselves to what is prescribed No. 53, and following.

59. The instructor will cause to be executed, marching in retreat, all that is prescribed for marching in advance; the commands and the means of execution will be the same.

60. The instructor having halted the company, will, when he may wish, cause it to face to the front by the commands prescribed, No. 62. The captain, the covering sergeant, and the directing sergeant, will resume their habitual places in the line, the moment they shall have faced about.

61. The company being in march by the front rank, if the instructor should wish it to march in retreat, he will cause the right about to be executed while marching, and to this effect will command:

1. *Company.* 2. *Right about.* 3. MARCH.

62. At the third command, the company will promptly face about, and recommence the march by the rear rank.

63. The directing sergeant will face about with the company, and will move rapidly six paces in front of the file closers, and upon the prolongation of the guide. The instruc-

tor will plaçe him in the proper direction by the means prescribed, No. 52. The captain, the covering sergeant, and the men, will conform to the principles prescribed for the march in retreat.

64. When the instructor wishes the company to march by the front rank, he will give the same commands, and will regulate the direction of the march by the same means.

LESSON THIRD.

To march by the flank.

65. The company being in line of battle, and at a halt, when the instructor shall wish to cause it to march by the right flank, he will command:

1. *Company, right*—Face. 2. *Forward.*
3. March.

66. At the first command, the company will face to the right, the covering sergeant will place himself at the head of the front rank, the captain having stepped out for the purpose, so far as to find himself by the side

of the sergeant, and on his left; the front rank will double as is prescribed in the School of the Soldier, No. 144; the rear rank will, at the same time, side step to the right one pace, and double in the same manner; so that when the movement is completed, the files will be formed of four men aligned, and elbow to elbow. The intervals will be preserved.

67. The file closers will also move by side step to the right, so that when the ranks are formed, they will be two paces from the rearmost rank.

68. At the command *march*, the company will move off briskly in quick time; the covering sergeant at the head of the front rank, and the captain on his left, will march straight forward. The men of each file will march abreast of their respective front rank men, heads direct to the front; the file closers will march opposite their places in line of battle.

69. The instructor will cause the principles of the march by the flank to be observed, in placing himself, pending the march, as prescribed in the School of the Soldier, No. 147.

70. The instructor will cause the march by the left flank to be executed by the same com-

mands, substituting *left* for *right;* the ranks will double as has been prescribed in the school for the soldier, No. 146; the rear rank will side-step to the left one pace before doubling.

71. At the instant the company faces to the left, the left guide will place himself at the head of the front rank; the captain will pass rapidly to the left, and place himself by the right side of this guide; the covering sergeant will replace the captain in the front rank, the moment the latter quits it to go to the left.

LESSON FOURTH.

Article First.

To break into column by platoon, either at a halt or in march.

72. The company being at a halt, in line of battle, the instructor, wishing to break it into column, by platoon to the right, will command:

1. *By platoon, right wheel.* 2. March.

73. At the first command, the chiefs of platoons will rapidly place themselves two paces

before the centres of their respective platoons, the lieutenant passing around the left of the company. They need not occupy themselves with dressing, one upon the other. The covering sergeant will replace the captain in the front rank.

74. At the command *march*, the right front rank man of each platoon will face to the right, the covering sergeant standing fast; the chief of each platoon will move quickly by the shortest line, a little beyond the point at which the marching flank will rest when the wheel shall be completed, face to the late rear, and place himself so that the line which he forms with the man on the right (who had faced), shall be perpendicular to that occupied by the company in line of battle; each platoon will wheel according to the principles prescribed for the wheel on a fixed pivot, and when the man who conducts the marching flank shall approach near to the perpendicular, its chief will command:

1. *Platoon.* 2. Halt.

75. At the command *halt*, which will be given at the instant the man who conducts

the marching flank shall have arrived at three paces from the perpendicular, the platoon will halt; the covering sergeant will move to the point where the left of the first platoon is to rest, passing by the front rank; the second sergeant will place himself, in like manner, in respect to the second platoon. Each will take care to leave between himself and the man on the right of his platoon, a space equal to its front; the captain and first lieutenant will look to this, and each take care to align the sergeant between himself and the man of the platoon who had faced to the right.

76. The guide of each platoon being thus established on the perpendicular, each chief will place himself two paces outside of his guide, and facing towards him, will command:

3. *Left*—Dress.

77. The alignment being ended, each chief of platoon will command, Front, and place himself two paces before its centre.

78. The file closers will conform themselves to the movement of their respective platoons, preserving always the distance of two paces from the rear rank.

79. The company will break by platoon to the left, according to the same principles. The instructor will command:

1. *By platoon, left wheel.* 2. MARCH.

80. The first command will be executed in the same manner as if breaking by platoon to the right.

81. At the command *march*, the left front rank man of each platoon will face to the left, and the platoons will wheel to the left, according to the principles prescribed for the wheel on a fixed pivot; the chiefs of platoon will conform to the principles indicated Nos. 73 and 76.

82. At the command *halt*, given by the chief of each platoon, the covering sergeant on the right of the front rank of the first platoon, and the second sergeant near the left of the second platoon, will each move to the points where the right of his platoon is to rest. The chief of each platoon should be careful to align the sergeant between himself and the man of the platoon who had faced to the left, and will then command:

Right—DRESS.

83. The platoons being aligned, each chief of platoon will command, FRONT, and place himself opposite its centre.

84. The instructor wishing to break the company by platoon to the right, and to move the column forward after the wheel is completed, will caution the company to that effect, and command:

1. *By Platoon, right wheel.* 2. MARCH.

85. At the first command, the chiefs of platoon will move rapidly in front of their respective platoons, conforming to what has been prescribed, No. 73, and will remain in this position during the continuance of the wheel. The covering sergeant will replace the chief of the first platoon in the front rank.

86. At the command *march*, the platoons will wheel to the right, conforming to the principles herein described; the man on the pivot will not face to the right, but will mark time, conforming himself to the movement of the marching flank; and when the man who is on the left of this flank shall arrive near

the perpendicular, the instructor will command:

3. *Forward.* 4. MARCH. 5. *Guide left.*

87. At the fourth command, which will be given at the instant the wheel is completed, the platoons will move straight to the front, all the men taking the step of twenty-eight inches. The covering sergeant and the second sergeant will move rapidly to the left of their respective platoons, the former passing before the front rank. The leading guide will immediately take points on the ground in the direction which may be indicated to him by the instructor.

88. At the fifth command, the men will take the touch of elbows lightly to the left.

89. If the guide of the second platoon should lose his distance, or the line of direction, he will conform to the principles herein prescribed, Nos. 75 and 76.

90. If the company be marching in line to the front, the instructor will cause it to break by platoons to the right by the same commands. At the command *march*, the platoons will wheel in the manner already ex-

plained; the man on the pivot will take care to mark time in his place, without advancing or receding; the instructor, the chiefs of platoon, and the guides, will conform to what has been prescribed, Nos. 77 and following.

91. The company may be broken by platoons to the left, according to the same principles, and by inverse means, the instructor giving the commands prescribed, Nos. 73 and 74, substituting *left* for *right*, and reciprocally.

92. The movements explained in Nos. 84 and 90 will only be executed after the company has become well established in the principles of the march in column, Articles Second and Third.

Article Second.

To march in column.

93. The company having broken by platoon, right (or left) in front, the instructor, wishing to cause the column to march, will throw himself twenty-five or thirty paces to the front, face to the guides, place himself correctly on their direction, and caution the leading guide to take points on the ground.

94. The instructor being thus placed, the guide of the leading platoon will take two points on the ground in the straight line passing between his own and the heels of the instructor.

95. These dispositions made, the instructor will step aside and command:

1. *Column forward.* 2. *Guide left* (or *right*). 3. MARCH.

96. At the command *march*, promptly repeated by the chiefs of platoons, they, as well as the guides, will lead off, by a decided step, their respective platoons, in order that the whole may move smartly, and at the same moment.

97. The men will each feel lightly the elbow of his neighbor towards the guide, and conform himself, in marching, to the principles prescribed in the School of the Soldier, No. 70. The man next to the guide, in each platoon, will take care never to pass him, and also to march always about six inches to the right (or left) from him, in order not to push him out of the direction.

98. The leading guide will observe, with the greatest precision, the length and cadence of the step, and maintain the direction of his march by the means prescribed No. 119:

99. The following guide will march exactly in the trace of the leading one, preserving between the latter and himself a distance precisely equal to the front of his platoon, and marching in the same step with the leading guide.

100. If the following guide lose his distance from the one leading (which can only happen by his own fault), he will correct himself by slightly lengthening or shortening a few steps, in order that there may not be sudden quickenings or slackenings in the march of his platoon.

101. If the same guide, having neglected to march exactly in the trace of the preceding one, find himself sensibly out of the direction, he will remedy this fault by advancing more or less the shoulder opposite to the true direction, and thus, in a few steps, insensibly regain it, without the inconvenience of the oblique step, which would cause a loss of distance. In all cases, each chief of platoon will cause it to conform to the movements of its guide.

LESSON FIFTH.

To break the company into platoons, and to re-form the company.

To break the company into platoons.

102. The company marching in the cadenced step, and supposed to make part of a column, right in front, when the instructor shall wish to cause it to break by platoon, he will give the order to the captain, who will command: 1. *Break into platoons*, and immediately place himself before the centre of the first platoon.

103. At the command *break into platoons*, the first lieutenant will pass quickly around the left to the centre of his platoon, and give the caution: *Mark time.*

104. The captain will then command: 2. *March.*

105. The first platoon will continue to march straight forward; the covering sergeant will move rapidly to the left flank of his platoon (passing by the front rank) as soon as the flank shall be disengaged.

106. At the command *march*, given by the captain, the second platoon will begin to mark time; its chief will immediately add: 1. *Right oblique;* 2. MARCH. The last command will be given so that this platoon may commence obliquing the instant the rear rank of the first platoon shall have passed. The men will shorten the step in obliquing, so that when the command *forward march*, is given, the platoon may have its exact distance.

107. The guide of the second platoon being near the direction of the guide of the first, the chief of the second will command *Forward*, and add MARCH, the instant that the guide of his platoon shall cover the guide of the first.

108. In a column, left in front, the company will break into platoons by inverse means, applying to the first platoon all that has been prescribed for the second, and reciprocally.

109. In this case the left guide of the company will shift to the right flank of the second platoon, and the covering sergeant will remain on the right of the first.

To re-form the company.

110. The column, by platoon, being in march, right in front, when the instructor shall wish to cause it to form company, he will give the order to the captain, who will command: *Form company.*

111. Having given this command, the captain will immediately add: 1. *First platoon;* 2. *Right oblique.*

112. The chief of the second platoon will caution it to continue to march straight forward.

113. The captain will then command: 3. MARCH.

114. At this command, repeated by the chief of the second, the first platoon will oblique to the right, in order to unmask the second; the covering sergeant, on the left of the first platoon will return to the right of the company, passing by the front rank.

115. When the first platoon shall have nearly unmasked the second, the captain will command: 1. *Mark time*, and at the instant the unmasking shall be complete, he will add: 2. MARCH. The first platoon will then cease to oblique, and mark time.

116. In the mean time the second platoon will have continued to march straight forward, and when it shall be nearly up with the first, the captain will command *Forward*, and at the instant the two platoons shall unite, add MARCH; the first platoon will then cease to mark time.

117. In a column, left in front, the same movement will be executed by inverse means, the chief of the second platoon giving the command *Forward*, and the captain adding the command MARCH, when the platoons are united.

118. The guide of the second platoon on its right, will pass to its left flank the moment the platoon begins to oblique; the guide of the first on its right, remaining on that flank of the platoon.

119. The instructor will also sometimes cause the company to break and re-form, by platoon, by his own direct command. In this case he will give the general commands prescribed for the captain above: 1. *Break into platoons;* 2. MARCH; and, 1. *Form company;* 2. MARCH.

120. If, in breaking the company into pla-

toons, the sub-division that breaks off should mark time too long, it might, in a column of many sub-divisions, arrest the march of the following one, which would cause a lengthening of the column, and a loss of distances.

121. In breaking into platoons, it is necessary that the platoons which oblique should not shorten the step too much, in order not to lose distance in column, and not to arrest the march of the following sub-division.

122. If a platoon obliques too far to a flank, it would be obliged to oblique again to the opposite flank, to regain the direction, and by the double movement arrest, probably, the march of the following sub-division.

123. The chiefs of those platoons which oblique will face to their platoons, in order to enforce the observance of the foregoing principles.

124. When, in a column of several companies, they break in succession, it is of the greatest importance that each company should continue to march in the same step, without shortening or slackening, whilst that which precedes breaks, although the following company should close up on the preceding one.

This attention is essential to guard against an elongation of the column.

125. Faults of but little moment, in a column of a few companies, would be serious inconveniences in a general column of many battalions. Hence the instructor will give the greatest care in causing all the prescribed principles to be strictly observed. To this end he will hold himself on the directing flank, the better to observe all the movements.

Being in column, to break files to the rear, and to cause them to re-enter into line.

126. The company being in march, and supposed to constitute a sub-division of a column, right (or left) in front, when the instructor shall wish to cause files to break off, he will give the order to the captain, who will immediately turn to his company, and command:

1. *Two files from left* (or *right*) *to rear.*
2. MARCH.

127. At the command *march*, the two files on the left (or right) of the company will mark

time, the others will continue to march straight forward; the two rear rank men of these files will, as soon as the rear rank of the company shall clear them, move to the right by advancing the outer shoulder; the odd number will place himself behind the third file from that flank, the even number behind the fourth, passing for this purpose behind the odd number; the two front rank men will, in like manner, move to the right, when the rear rank of the company shall clear them; the odd number will place himself behind the first file, the even number behind the second file, passing for this purpose behind the odd number. If the files are broken from the right, the men will move to the left, advancing the outer shoulder, the even number of the rear rank will place himself behind the third file, the odd number of the second rank behind the fourth; the even number of the front rank behind the first file, the odd number of the same rank behind the second, the odd numbers for this purpose passing behind the even numbers. The men will be careful not to lose their distances, and to keep aligned.

128. If the instructor should still wish to break two files from the same side, he will give the order to the captain, who will proceed as above directed.

129. At the command *march*, given by the captain, the files already broken, advancing a little the outer shoulder, will gain the space of two files to the right, if the files are broken from the left, and to the left, if the files are broken from the right, shortening, at the same time, the step, in order to make room between themselves and the rear rank of the company for the files last ordered to the rear; the latter will break by the same commands and in the same manner as the first. The men who double should increase the length of the step in order to prevent distances from being lost.

130. The instructor may thus diminish the front of a company by breaking off successive groups of two files, but the new files must always be broken from the same side.

131. The instructor, wishing to cause files broken off to return into line, will give the order to the captain, who will immediately command:

1. *Two files into line.* 2. MARCH.

132. At the command *march*, the first two files of those marching by the flank will return briskly into line, and the other will gain the space of two files by advancing the inner shoulder towards the flank to which they belong.

133. The captain will turn to his company, to watch the observance of the principles which have just been prescribed.

134. The instructor having caused groups of two files to break one after another, and to return again into line, will afterwards cause two or three groups to break together; and for this purpose will command: *Four or six files from the left* (or *right*) *to rear;* MARCH. The files designated will mark time; each rank will advance a little the outer shoulder as soon as the rear rank of the company shall clear it, will oblique at once, and each group will place itself behind the four neighboring files, and in the same manner, as if the movement had been executed group by group, taking care that the distances are preserved.

135. The instructor will next order the captain to cause two or three groups to be brought into line at once, who, turning to the company, will command:

Four or six files into line—MARCH.

136. At the command *march*, the files designated will advance the inner shoulder, move up and form on flank of the company by the shortest lines.

137. As often as files shall break off to the rear, the guide on that flank will gradually close on the nearest front rank man remaining in line, and he will also open out to make room for files ordered into line.

138. The files which march in the rear are disposed in the following order: the left files as if the company was marching by the right flank, and the right files as if the company was marching by the left flank. Consequently, whenever there is on the right or left of a sub-division, a file which does not belong to a group, it will be broken singly.

139. It is necessary to the preservation of distances in column that the men should be habituated in the school of details to exe-

cute the movements of this article with precision.

140. If new files broken off do not step well to the left or right in obliquing; if, when files are ordered into line, they do not move up with promptitude and precision, in either case the following files will be arrested in their march, and thereby cause the column to be lengthened out.

141. The instructor will place himself on the flank from which the files are broken, to assure himself of the exact observance of the principles.

142. Files will only be broken off from the side of direction, in order that the whole company may easily pass from the front to the flank march.

Formation of a company from two ranks into single rank, and reciprocally.

143. The company being formed into two ranks in the manner indicated, No. 8, School of the Soldier, and supposed to make part of a column, right or left in front, when the instructor shall wish to form it into single rank, he will command:

1. *In one rank, form company.* 2. MARCH.

144. At the first command, the right guide will face to the right.

145. At the command *march*, the right guide will step off and march in the prolongation of the front rank.

146. The first file will step off at the same time with the guide; the front rank man will turn to the right at the first step, follow the guide, and be himself followed by the rear rank man of his file, who will come to turn on the same spot where he had turned. The second file, and successively all the other files, will step off as has been prescribed for the first, the front rank man of each file following immediately the rear rank man of the file next on his right. The captain will superintend the movement, and when the last man shall have stepped off, he will halt the company, and face it to the front.

147. The file closers will take their places in line of battle, two paces in rear of the rank.

148. The company being in single rank, when the instructor shall wish to form it into two ranks, he will command:

1. *In two ranks, form company.* 2. *Company right*—Face. 3. March.

149. At the second command, the company will face to the right: the right guide and the man on the right will remain faced to the front.

150. At the command *march*, the men who have faced to the right will step off, and form files in the following manner: the second man in the rank will place himself behind the first to form the first file; the third will place himself by the side of the first in the front rank; the fourth behind the third in the rear rank. All the others will, in like manner, place themselves, alternately, in the front and rear rank, and will thus form files of two men, on the left of those already formed.

151. The formations above described will be habitually executed by the right of companies; but when the instructor shall wish to have them executed by the left, he will face the company *about*, and post the guides in the rear rank.

152. The formation will then be executed by the same commands, and according to the

same principles as by the front rank; the movement commencing with the left file, now become the right, and in each file by the rear rank man, now become the front; the left guide will conform to what has been prescribed for the right.

153. The formation ended, the instructor will face the company to its proper front.

154. When a battalion in line has to execute either of the formations above described, the colonel will cause it to break to the rear by the right or left of companies, and will then give the commands just prescribed for the instructor. Each company will execute the movement as if acting singly.

Formation of a company from two ranks into four, and reciprocally, at a halt, and in march.

155. The company being formed in two ranks, at a halt, and supposed to form part of a column right in front, when the instructor shall wish to form it into four ranks, he will command:

1. *In four ranks, form company.* 2. *Company left*—FACE. 3. MARCH (or *double quick*—MARCH).

156. At the second command, the left guide will remain faced to the front, the company will face to the left: the rear rank will gain the distance of one pace from the front rank by a side step to the left and rear, and the men will form into four ranks, as prescribed in the School of the Soldier.

157. At the command *march*, the first file of four men will reface to the front without undoubling. All the other files of four will step off, and closing successively to about five inches of the preceding file, will halt, and immediately face to the front, the men remaining doubled.

158. The file closers will take their new places in line of battle, at two paces in rear of the fourth rank.

159. The captain will superintend the movement.

160. The company being in four ranks, when the instructor shall wish to form it into two ranks, he will command :

1. *In two ranks, form company.* 2. *Company right*—FACE. 3. MARCH (or *double quick*—MARCH).

161. At the second command the left guide will stand fast, the company will face to the right.

162. At the command *march*, the right guide will step off and march in the prolongation of the front rank. The leading file of four men will step off at the same time, the other files standing fast; the second file will step off when there shall be between it and the first space sufficient to form into two ranks. The following files will execute successively what has been prescribed for the second. As soon as the last file shall have its distance, the instructor will command:

1. *Company.* 2. HALT. 3. FRONT.

163. At the command *front*, the company will face to the front, and the files will undouble.

164. The company being formed in two ranks, and marching to the front, when the

instructor shall wish to form it into four ranks, he will command:

1. *In four ranks, form company.* 2. *By the left, double files.* 3. MARCH (or *double quick*—MARCH).

165. At the command *march*, the left guide and the left file of the company will continue to march straight to the front: the company will make a half face to the left, the odd numbers placing themselves behind the even numbers. The even numbers of the rear rank will shorten their steps a little, to permit the odd numbers of the front rank to get between them and the even numbers of that rank. The files thus formed of fours, except the left file, will continue to march obliquely, lengthening their steps slightly, so as to keep constantly abreast of the guide; each file will close successively on the file next on its left, and when at the proper distance from that file, will face to the front by a half face to the right, and take the touch of elbows to the left.

166. The company being in march to the front in four ranks, when the instructor shall

wish to form it into two ranks, he will command:

1. *In two ranks, form company.* 2. *By the right, undouble files.* 3. MARCH (or *double quick*—MARCH).

167. At the command *march*, the left guide and the left file of the company will continue to march straight to the front; the company will make a half face to the right, and march obliquely, lengthening the step a little, in order to keep as near as possible abreast of the guide. As soon as the second file from the left shall have gained to the right the interval necessary for the left file to form into two ranks, the second file will face to the front by a half face to the left, and march straight forward; the left file will immediately form into two ranks, and take the touch of elbows to the left. Each file will execute successively what has just been prescribed for the file next to the left, and each file will form into two ranks when the file next on its right has obliqued the required distance, and faced to the front.

168. If the company be supposed to make part of a column, left in front, these different movements will be executed according to the same principles, and by inverse means, substituting the indication *left* for *right*.

SCHOOL OF THE BATTALION.

General Rules and Divisions of the School of the Battalion.

1. This school has for it object the instruction of battalions singly, and thus prepare them for manœuvres in line. The harmony so indispensable in the movements of many battalions can only be attained by the use of the same commands, the same principles, and the same means of execution. Hence, all colonels, and actual commanders of battalions will conform themselves, without addition or curtailment, to what will herein be prescribed.

2. When a battalion instructed in this drill shall manœuvre in line, the colonel will regulate its movements, as prescribed in the third volume of the Tactics for Heavy Infantry.

3. The School of the Battalion will be divided into five parts.

4. The first will comprehend opening and closing ranks, and the execution of the different fires.

5. The second, the different modes of passing from the order in battle to the order in column.

6. The third, the march in column, and the other movements incident thereto.

7. The fourth, the different modes of passing from the order in column to the order in battle.

8. The fifth will comprehend the march in line of battle, in advance and in retreat; the passage of defiles in retreat; the march by the flank, the formation by file into line of battle; the change of front; the column doubled on the centre; dispositions against cavalry; the rally, and rules for manœuvering by the rear rank.

PART FIRST.

Opening and closing ranks, and the execution of the different fires.

To open and to close ranks.

9. The colonel, wishing the ranks to be opened, will command:

1. *Prepare to open ranks.*

10. At this command, the lieutenant-colonel and major will place themselves on the right of the battalion, the first on the flank of the file closers, and the second four paces from the front rank of the battalion.

11. These dispositions being made, the colonel will command:

2. *To the rear, open order.* 3. MARCH.

12. At the second command, the covering sergeants, and the sergeants on the left of the battalion, will place themselves four paces in rear of the front rank, and opposite their places in the line of battle, in order to mark the new alignment of the rear rank; they will be aligned by the major on the left sergeant of the battalion, who will be careful to place himself exactly four paces in rear of the front rank, and to hold his piece between the eyes, erect and inverted, the better to indicate to the major the direction to be given to the covering sergeants.

13. At the command *march*, the rear rank

and the file closers will step to the rear without counting steps; the men will pass a little in rear of the line traced by this rank, halt, and dress forward on the covering sergeants, who will align correctly the men of their respective companies.

14. The file closers will fall back and preserve the distance of two paces from the rear rank, glancing eyes to the right; the lieutenant-colonel will, from the right, align them on the file closer of the left, who, having placed himself accurately two paces from the rear rank, will invert his piece, and hold it up erect between his eyes, the better to be seen by the lieutenant-colonel.

15. The colonel, seeing the ranks aligned, will command:

4. FRONT.

At this command, the lieutenant-colonel, major, and the left sergeant, will retake their places in line of battle.

16. The colonel will cause the ranks to be closed by the commands prescribed for the instructor in the School of the Company, No. 28.

PART SECOND.

Different modes of passing from the order of battle to the order in column.

ARTICLE FIRST.

To break to the right or the left into column.

17. Lines of battle will habitually break into column by company; they may also break by division or by platoon.

18. It is here supposed that the colonel wishes to break by company to the right; he will command:

1. *By company, right wheel.* 2. MARCH (or *double quick*—MARCH).

19. At the first command, each captain will place himself rapidly before the centre of his company, and caution it that it has to wheel to the right; each covering sergeant will replace his captain in the front rank.

20. At the command *march*, each company will break to the right, according to the principles prescribed in the School of the Com-

pany, No. 173; each captain will conform himself to what is prescribed for the chiefs of platoon; the left guide, as soon as he can pass, will place himself on the left of the front rank to conduct the marching flank, and when he shall have approached near to the perpendicular, the captain will command: 1. *Such company.* 2. HALT.

21. At the second command, which will be given at the instant the left guide shall be at the distance of three paces from the perpendicular, the company will halt; the guide will advance and place his left arm lightly against the breast of the captain, who will establish him on the alignment of the man who has faced to the right; the covering sergeant will place himself correctly on the alignment on the right of that man; which being executed, the captain will align his company by the left, command FRONT, and place himself two paces before its centre.

22. The captains having commanded FRONT, the guides, although some of them may not be in the direction of the preceding guides, will stand fast, in order that the error of a company that has wheeled too much or too

little may not be propagated; the guides not in the direction will readily come into it when the column is put in march.

23. A battalion in line of battle will break into column by company to the left, according to the same principles, and by inverse means; the covering sergeant of each company will conduct the marching flank, and the left guide will place himself on the left of the front rank at the moment the company halts.

24. When the battalion breaks by division, the indication *division* will be substituted in the commands for that of *company;* the chief of each division (the senior captain) will conform himself to what is prescribed for the chief of company, and will place himself two paces before the centre of his division; the junior captain, if not already there, will place himself in the interval between the two companies in the front rank, and be covered by the covering sergeant of the left company in the rear rank. The right guide of the right company will be the right guide, and the left guide of the left company, the left guide of the division.

25. When the battalion shall break by pla-

toon to the right or to the left, each first lieutenant will pass around the left of his company to place himself in front of the second platoon, and for this purpose, each covering sergeant, except the one of the right company, will step, for the moment, in rear of the right file of his company.

26. When the battalion breaks by division to the right, and there is an odd company, the captain of this company (the left), after wheeling into column, will cause it to oblique to the left, halt it at company distance from the preceding division, place his left guide on the direction of the column, and then align his company by the left. When the line breaks by division to the left, the odd company will be in front; its captain, having wheeled it into column, will cause it to oblique to the right, halt it at a division distance from the division next in the rear, place his right guide on the direction of the other guides, and align the company by the right.

27. When the colonel shall wish to move the column forward without halting it, he will caution the battalion to that effect, and command:

1. *By company, right wheel.* 2. MARCH (*or double quick*—MARCH.)

28. At the first command, the captains of companies will execute what is prescribed for breaking into column from a halt.

29. At the second command, they will remain in front of their companies to superintend the movement; the companies will wheel to the right on fixed pivots, as indicated in the School of the Company, No. 185; the left guides will conform to what is prescribed above; when they shall arrive near the perpendicular, the colonel will command:

3. *Forward.* 4. MARCH. 5. *Guide left.*

30. At the third command, each covering sergeant will place himself by the right side of the man on the right of the front rank of his company. At the fourth command, which will be given at the instant the wheel is completed, the companies will cease to wheel and march straight forward. At the fifth, the men will take the touch of elbows to the left.

The leading guide will march in the direction indicated to him by the lieutenant-colonel. The guides will immediately conform themselves to the principles of the march, in column, School of the Company, No. 200, and following.

31. If the battalion be marched in line of battle, the colonel will cause it to wheel to the right or left, by the same commands and the same means; but he should previously caution the battalion that it is to continue the march.

32. A battalion in line of battle will break into column by company to the left, according to the same principles and by inverse means; the covering sergeant of each company will conduct the marching flank, and the left guides will place themselves on the left of their respective companies at the command *forward.*

ARTICLE SECOND.

To break to the rear, by the right or left, into column, and to advance or retire by the right or left of companies.

23. When the colonel shall wish to cause the battalion to break to the rear, by the right, into column by company, he will command :

1. *By the right of companies to the rear into column.* 2. *Battalion right*—FACE. 3. MARCH (*or double quick*—MARCH.)

34. At the first command, each captain will place himself before the centre of his company, and caution it to face to the right, the covering sergeant will step into the front rank.

35. At the second command, the battalion will face to the right; each captain will hasten to the right of his company, and break two files to the rear; the first file will break the whole depth of the two ranks; the second file less; which being executed, the captain will place himself so that his breast may touch lightly the left arm of the front rank man of the last file in the company next on the right of his own. The captain of the right company will place himself as if there were a company on his right, and will align himself on the other captains. The covering sergeant of each company will break to the rear with the right files, and place himself before the front rank of the first file, to conduct him.

36. At the command *march*, the first file of each company will wheel to the right; the

covering sergeant, placed before this file, will conduct it perpendicularly to the rear. The other files will come successively to wheel on the same spot. The captains will stand fast, see their companies file past, and at the instant the last file shall have wheeled, each captain will command:

1. *Such Company.* 2. HALT. 3. FRONT.
4. *Left*—DRESS.

37. At the instant the company faces to the front, its left guide will place himself so that his left arm may touch lightly the breast of his captain.

38. At the fourth command, the company will align itself on its left guide, the captain so directing it, that the new alignment may be perpendicular to that which the company had occupied in line of battle, and the better to judge this, he will step back two paces from the flank.

39. The company being aligned, the captain will command: FRONT, and take his place before its centre.

40. The battalion marching in line of battle,

when the colonel shall wish to break into column by company to the rear, by the right, he will command:

1. *By the right of companies to the rear into column.* 2. *Battalion, by the right flank.* 3. MARCH (or *double quick*—MARCH).

41. At the first command, each captain will step briskly in front of the centre of his company, and caution it to face *by the right flank.*

42. At the command *march*, the battalion will face to the right; each captain will move rapidly to the right of his company and cause it to break to the right; the first file of each company will wheel to the right, and the covering sergeant placed in front of this file will conduct it perpendicularly to the rear; the other files will wheel successively at the same place as the first. The captains will see their companies file past them; when the last files have wheeled, the colonel will command:

3. *Battalion, by the left flank*—MARCH. 4. *Guide left.*

43. At the command *march*, the companies

will face to the left, and march in column in the new direction. The captains will place themselves in front of the centres of their respective companies. At the fourth command, the guides will conform to the principles of the march in column; the leading one will move in the direction indicated to him by the lieutenant-colonel. The men will take the touch of elbows to the left.

44. To break to the rear by the left, the colonel will give the same command as in the case of breaking to the rear by the right, substituting the indication *left*, for that of *right*.

45. The movement will be executed according to the same principles. Each captain will hasten to the left of his company, cause the first two files to break to the rear, and then place his breast against the right file of the company next on the left of his own, in the manner prescribed above.

46. As soon as the two files break to the rear, the left guide of each company will place himself before the front rank man of the headmost file, to conduct him.

47. The instant the companies face to the front, the right guide of each will place him-

self so that his right arm may lightly touch the breast of his captain.

48. The battalion may be broken by division to the rear, by the right or left, in like manner in this case, the indication *divisions* will be substituted, in the first command, for that of *companies;* the chiefs of division will conform themselves to what is prescribed for the chiefs of company. The junior captain in each division will place himself, when the division faces to a flank, by the side of the covering sergeant of the left company, who steps into the front rank.

49. If there be an odd number of companies and the battalion breaks by division to the rear, whether by the right or left, the captain of the left company will conform to what is prescribed, No. 77.

50. This manner of breaking into column being at once the most prompt and regular, will be preferred on actual service, unless there be some particular reason for breaking to the front.

51. If the battalion be in line and at a halt, and the colonel should wish to advance or retire by the right of companies, he will command:

1. *By the right of companies to the front* (or *rear*). 2. *Battalion, right*—FACE. 3. MARCH (or *double quick*—MARCH). 4. *Guide right* (*left*) or (*centre*).

52. At the first command, each captain will move rapidly two paces in front of the centre of his company, and caution it to face to the right; the covering sergeants will replace the captains in the front rank.

53. At the second command, the battalion will face to the right, and each captain moving quickly to the right of his company will cause files to break to the front, according to the principles indicated, No. 89.

54. At the command *march*, each captain placing himself on the left of his leading guide will conduct his company perpendicularly to the original line. At the fourth command, the guide of each company will dress to the right, left, or centre, according to the indication given, taking care to preserve accurately his distance.

55. If the colonel should wish to move to the front, or rear, by the left of companies,

the movement will be executed by the same means and the same commands, substituting *left* for *right.*

56. If the battalion be in march, and the colonel should wish to advance or retire by the right of companies, he will command:

1. *By the right of companies to the front* (or *rear*). 2. *Battalion, by the right flank.* 3. MARCH (or *double quick* — MARCH). 4. *Guide right* (*left*) or (*centre*).

57. Which will be executed according to the principles and means prescribed, Nos. 95 and following, and 106 and following. At the first command, the color and general guides will take their places as in column.

58. If the colonel should wish to advance or retire by the left of companies, the movement will be executed by the same means and the same commands, substituting *left* for *right.*

59. If the battalion be advancing by the right or left of companies, and the colonel should wish to form line to the front, he will command:

1. *By companies into line.* 2. MARCH (or *double quick*—MARCH). 3. *Guide centre.*

60. At the command *march*, briskly repeated by the captains, each company will be formed into line, as prescribed in the School of the Company, No. 154.

61. At the third command, the color and general guides will move rapidly to their places in line, as will be hereinafter prescribed, No. 405.

62. If the battalion be retiring by the right or left of companies, and the colonel should wish to form line facing the enemy, he will first cause the companies to face about while marching, and immediately form in line by the commands and means prescribed, No. 113 and following.

To ploy the battalion into close column.

63. This movement may be executed by company or by division, on the right or left sub-division, or on any other sub-division, right or left in front.

64. The examples in this school will sup-

pose the presence of four divisions, with directions for an odd company; but what will be prescribed for four, will serve equally for two, three, or five divisions.

65. To ploy the battalion into close column by division in rear of the first, the colonel will command:

1. *Close column, by division.* 2. *On the first division, right in front.* 3. *Battalion, right* —FACE. 4. MARCH (*or double quick*—MARCH).

66. At the second command, all the chiefs of division will place themselves before the centres of their divisions; the chief of the first will caution it to stand fast; the chiefs of the three others will remind them that they will have to face to the right, and the covering sergeant of the right company of each division will replace his captain in the front rank, as soon as the latter steps out.

67. At the third command, the last three divisions will face to the right; the chief of each division will hasten to its right, and cause files to be broken to the rear, as indicated No. 89; the right guide will break at

the same time, and place himself before the front rank man of the first file, to conduct him, and each chief of division will place himself by the side of this guide.

68. The moment these divisions face to the right, the junior captain in each will place himself on the left of the covering sergeant of the left company, who will place himself in the front rank. *This rule is general for all the ployments by division.*

69. At the command *march*, the chief of the first division will add, *guide left;* at this, its left guide will place himself on its left, as soon as the movement of the second division may permit, and the file closers will advance one pace upon the rear rank.

70. All the other divisions, each conducted by its chief, will step off together, to take their places in the column; the second will gain, in wheeling by file to the rear, the space of six paces, which ought to separate its guide from the guide of the first division, and so direct its march as to enter the column on a line parallel to this division; the third and fourth divisions will direct themselves diagonally towards, but a

little in rear of, the points at which they ought, respectively, to enter the column; at six paces from the left flank of the column, the head of each of these divisions will incline a little to the left, in order to enter the column as has just been prescribed for the second, taking care also to leave the distance of six paces between its guide and the guide of the preceding division. At the moment the divisions put themselves in march to enter the column, the file closers of each will incline to the left so as to bring themselves to the distance of a pace from the rear rank.

71. Each chief of these three divisions will conduct his division till he shall be up with the guide of the directing one; the chief will then himself halt, see his division file past, and halt it the instant the last file shall have passed, commanding: 1. *Such division*; 2. HALT; 3. FRONT; 4. *Left*—DRESS.

72. At the second command, the division will halt; the left guide will place himself promptly on the direction, six paces from the guide which precedes him, in order that, the column being formed, the divisions may be separated the distance of four paces.

73. At the third command, the division will face to the front; at the fourth, it will be aligned by its chief, who will place himself two paces outside of his guide, and direct the alignment so that his division may be parallel to that which precedes—which being done, he will command, FRONT, and place himself before the centre of his division.

74. If any division, after the command *front*, be not at its proper distance, and this can only happen through the negligence of its chief, such division will remain in its place, in order that the fault may not be propagated.

75. The movement being ended, the colonel will command:

Guides, about—FACE.

76. At this, the guides who are faced to the rear, will face to the front.

77. To ploy the battalion in rear, or in front of the fourth division, the colonel will command:

1. *Close column by division.* 2. *On the fourth division, left* (or *right*) *in front.* 3. *Battalion, left*—FACE. 4. MARCH (or *double quick*—MARCH).

78. These movements will be executed according to the principles of those which precede, but by inverse means: the fourth division on which the battalion ploys will stand fast; the instant the movement commences, its chief will command, *guide right* (or *left*).

79. The foregoing examples embrace all the principles: thus, when the colonel shall wish to ploy the battalion on an interior division, he will command:

1. *Close column by division.* 2. *On such division, right* (or *left*) *in front.* 3. *Battalion inwards* — FACE. 4. MARCH (or *double quick*—MARCH).

80. The instant the movement commences, the chief of the directing division will command, *guide left* (or *right*).

81. The divisions, which, in the order in

battle, are to the right of the directing division, will face to the left; those which are to the left will face to the right.

82. If the right is to be in front, the right division will ploy in front of the directing division, and the left in its rear; the reverse, if the left is to be in front. And in all the foregoing suppositions, the division or divisions contiguous to the directing one, in wheeling by file to the front or rear, will gain the space of six paces, which ought to separate their guides from the guide of the directing division.

83. In the ployments on an interior division, the lieutenant-colonel will assure the positions of the guides in front, and the major those in rear of the directing division.

84. If the battalion be in march, instead of at a halt, the movement will be executed by combining the two gaits of quick and double quick time, and always in the rear of one ot the flank divisions.

85. The battalion being in march, to ploy it in rear of the first division, the colonel will command:

1. *Close column by division.* 2. *On the first division.* 3. *Battalion—by the right flank.* 4. *Double quick*—MARCH.

86. At the second command, each chief of division will move rapidly before the centre of his division and caution it to face to the right.

87. The chief of the first division will caution it to continue to march to the front, and he will command: *Quick march.*

88. At the command *march*, the chief of the first division will command: *Guide left.* At this, the left guide will move to the left flank of the division and direct himself on the point indicated.

89. The three other divisions will face to the right and move off in double quick time, breaking to the right to take their places in column; each chief of division will move rapidly to the right of his division in order to conduct it. The files will be careful to preserve their distances, and to march with a uniform and decided step. The color-bearer and general guides will retake their places in the ranks.

90. The second division will immediately enter the column, marching parallel to the first division; its chief will allow it to file past him, and when the last file is abreast of him, will command: 1. *Second division, by the left flank*—MARCH. 2. *Guide left*, and place himself in front of the centre of his division.

91. At the command *march*, the division will face to the left; at the second command, the left guide will march in the trace of the left guide of the first division; the men will take the touch of elbows to the left. When the second division has closed to its proper distance, its chief will command: *Quick time*—MARCH. This division will then change its step to quick time.

92. The chiefs of the third and fourth divisions will execute their movements according to the same principles, taking care to gain as much ground as possible towards the head of the column.

93. If the battalion had been previously marching in line at double quick time, when the fourth division shall have gained its distance, the colonel will command: *Double quick*—MARCH.

94. In this movement the lieutenant-colonel will move rapidly to the side of the leading guide, give him a point of direction, and then follow the movements of the first division. The major will follow the movement abreast with the left to the fourth division.

Remarks on ploying the battalion into column.

95. The battalion may be ployed into column at full, or half distance, on the same principles, and by the same commands, substituting for the first command: *Column at full* (or *half*) *distance by division.*

96. In the ployments and movements in columns, when the subdivisions execute the movements successively, such as—to take or close distances; to change direction by the flank of subdivisions, each chief of subdivision will cause his men to support arms after having aligned it and commanded, FRONT.

To march in column at full distance.

97. When the colonel shall wish to put the column into march, he will indicate to the

leading guide two distinct objects in front, on the line which the guide ought to follow. This guide will immediately put his shoulders in a square with that line, take the more distant object as the point of direction, and the nearer one as the intermediate point.

98. If only a single prominent object present itself in the direction the guide has to follow, he will face to it as before, and immediately endeavor to catch on the ground some intermediate point, by which to give steadiness to his march on the point of direction.

99. There being no prominent object to serve as the point of direction, the colonel will dispatch the lieutenant colonel or adjutant to place himself forty paces in advance, facing the column, and by a sign of the sword establish him on the direction he may wish to give to the leading guide; that officer being thus placed, this guide will take him as the point of direction, conforming himself to what is prescribed in the School of the Company, No. 87.

100. These dispositions being made, the colonel will command:

1. *Column forward.* 2. *Guide left* (or *right*). 3. MARCH (or *double quick*—MARCH).

101. At the command *march*, briskly repeated by the chiefs of subdivision, the column will put itself in march, conforming to what is prescribed in the School of the Company, No. 200 and following.

102. The leading guide may always maintain himself correctly on the direction by keeping steadily in view the two points indicated to him or chosen by himself; if these points have a certain elevation, he may be assured he is on the true direction, when the nearer masks the more distant point.

103. The following guides will preserve with exactness both step and distance; each will march in the trace of the guide who immediately precedes him, without occupying himself with the general direction.

104. The column being in march, the colonel will frequently cause the *about* to be executed while marching; to this effect, he will command:

1. *Battalion, right about.* 2. MARCH.
3. *Guide right.*

105. At the second command, the companies will face to the right about, and the column will then march forward in an opposite direction; the chiefs of subdivision will remain behind the front rank, the file closers in front of the rear rank, and the guides will place themselves in the same rank. The lieutenant-colonel will remain abreast of the first division, now in rear; the major will give a point of direction to the leading guide, and march abreast of him.

106. The colonel will hold himself habitually on the directing flank; he will look to the step and to the distances, and see that all the principles prescribed for the march in column, School of the Company, are observed.

107. These means, which the practice in that School ought to have rendered familiar, will give sufficient exactness to the direction of the column, and also enable it to form *forward* or *faced the rear*, *on the right*, or *on the left*, into line of battle, and *to close in mass*.

Remarks on the march in column.

108. Although the uncadenced step be that of columns in route marches, and also that which ought to be habitually employed in the *Evolutions of the Line*, because it leaves the men more at ease, and, consequently, is better adapted to movements on a large scale and to difficult grounds, nevertheless, as it is of paramount importance to confirm soldiers in the measure and the movement of the cadenced pace, the route step will be but little practised in the exercises by battalion, except in going to, and returning from, the ground of instruction, and for teaching the mechanism and movements of columns in route.

109. It is highly essential to the regularity of the march in column, that each guide follow exactly in the trace of the one immediately preceding, without occupying his attention with the general direction of the guides. If this principle be steadily observed, the guides will find themselves aligned, provided that the leading one march exactly in the direction indicated to him; and even should obstacles in his way force him into a momen-

tary deviation, the direction of the column would not necessarily be changed; whereas, if the following guides endeavor to conform themselves at once to all the movements of the leading one, in order to cover him in file, such endeavors would necessarily cause corresponding fluctuations in the column from right to left, and from left to right, and render the preservation of distances extremely difficult.

110. As a consequence of the principle, that *each guide shall exactly follow in the trace of the one who immediately precedes*, if, pending the march of the column, the colonel shall give a new point of direction, too near to the first to require a formal change of direction, the leading guide, advancing the one or other shoulder, will immediately direct himself on this point; the other guides will only conform themselves to this movement as each arrives at the point at which the first had executed it. Each subdivision will conform itself to the movements of its guide, the men insensibly lengthening or shortening the step, and advancing or refusing (throwing back) the shoulder opposite to the guide, but

without losing the touch of the elbow towards his side.

111. The column, by company, being in march, the colonel will cause it to diminish front by platoon, from front to rear, at once, and to increase front by platoon in like manner, which movements will be commanded and executed as prescribed in the School of the Company, Nos. 282 and 273 and following, changing the command *form company* to *form companies.* So may he increase and diminish, or diminish and increase front, according to the same principles, and at once by company, changing the command *form companies* to *form divisions*, and the command *break into platoons* to *break into companies.* In this case, the companies and divisions will execute what is prescribed for platoons and companies respectively.

To change direction in column at full distance.

112. The column being in march in the cadenced step, when the colonel shall wish to cause it to change direction, he will go to the point at which the change ought to be com-

menced, and establish a marker there, presenting the breast to the flank of the column; this marker, no matter to which side the change of direction is to be made, will be posted on the opposite side, and he will remain in position till the last subdivision of the battalion shall have passed. The leading subdivision being within a few paces of the marker the colonel will command.

Head of column to the left (or *right*).

113. At this, the chief of the leading subdivision will immediately take the guide on the side opposite the change of direction, if not already there. This guide will direct himself so as to graze the breast of the marker; arrived at this point, the chief will cause his subdivision to change direction by the commands and according to the principles prescribed in the School of the Company. When the wheel is completed, the chief of this subdivision will retake the guide if changed, on the side of the primitive direction.

114. The chief of each succeeding subdivision, as well as the guides, will conform to

what has just been explained for the leading subdivision.

115. The colonel will carefully see that the guide of each subdivision, in wheeling, does not throw himself without or within, but passes over all the points of the arc of the circle, which he ought to describe.

Remarks.

116. It has been demonstrated, School of the Company, how important it is, *first*, that each subdivision execute its change of direction precisely at the point where the leading one had changed, and that it arrive in a square with the direction; *second*, that the wheeling point ought, always, to be cleared in time, in order that the subdivision engaged in the wheel may not arrest the movement of the following one. The deeper the column, the more rigorously ought these principles to be observed; because, a fault that would be but slight in a column of a single battalion, would cause much embarrassment in one of great depth.

To halt the Column.

117. The column being in march, when the colonel shall wish to halt it, he will command:

1. *Column.* 2. HALT.

118. At the second command, briskly repeated by the captains, the column will halt; no guide will stir, though he may have lost his distance, or be out of the direction of the preceding guides.

119. The column being in march, in double quick time, will be halted by the same commands. At the command *halt*, the men will halt in their places, and will themselves rectify their positions in the ranks.

To close the column to half distance, or in mass.

120. A column by company being at full distance right in front, and at a halt, when the colonel shall wish to cause it to close to half distance, on the leading company, he will command:

1. *To half distance, close column.* 2. MARCH (or *double quick*—MARCH).

121. At the first command, the captain of the leading company will caution it to stand fast.

122. At the command *march*, which will be repeated by all the captains, except the captain of the leading company, this company will stand fast, and its chief will align it by the left; the file closers will close one pace upon the rear rank.

123. All the other companies will continue to march, and as each in succession arrives at platoon distance from the one which precedes, its captain will halt it.

124. At the instant that each company halts, its guide will place himself on the direction of the guides who precede, and the captain will align the company by the left; the file closers will close one pace upon the rear rank.

125. No particular attention need be given to the general direction of the guides before they respectively halt; it will suffice if each follow in the trace of the one who precedes him.

126. The colonel, on the side of the guides, will superintend the execution of the movement, observing that the captains hold their companies exactly at platoon distance the one from the other.

127. If the column be in march, the colonel will cause it to close by the same commands.

128. If the column be marching in double quick time, at the first command, the captain of the leading company will command *quick time*; the chiefs of the other companies will caution them to continue their march.

129. At the command *march*, the leading company will march in quick, and the other companies in double quick time; and as each arrives at platoon distance from the preceding one, its chief will cause it to march in quick time.

130. When the rearmost company shall have gained its distance, the colonel will command:

Double quick—MARCH.

131. When the colonel shall wish to halt the column, and to cause it to close at half distance at the same time, he will notify the captain of the leading company of his intention, who, at the command *march*, will halt his company, and align it by the left.

132. If the column be marching in quick time, and the colonel should not give the command *double quick*, the captain of the

leading company will halt his company at the command *march*, and align it by the left. In the case where the colonel adds the command *double quick*, the captains of companies will conform to what is prescribed, No. 262, and the movement will be executed as indicated, No. 263.

To close the column on the eighth, or rear-most company.

133. The column being at a halt, if instead of causing it to close at half distance on the first company, the colonel should wish to cause it to close on the eighth, he will command:

1. *On the eighth company, to half distance close column.* 2. *Battalion, about*—FACE. 3. *Column forward.* 4. *Guide right.* 5. MARCH (or *double quick*—MARCH).

134. At the second command, all the companies, except the eighth, will face about, and their guides will remain in the front rank, now the rear.

135. At the fourth command, all the cap-

tains will place themselves two paces outside of their companies on the directing flank.

136. At the command *march*, the eighth company will stand fast, and its captain will align it by the left; the other companies will put themselves in march, and, as each arrives at platoon distance from the one established before it, its captain will halt it, and face it to the front. At the moment that each company halts, the left guide, remaining faced to the rear, will place himself promptly on the direction of the guides already established. Immediately after, the captain will align his company by the left, and the file closers will close one pace on the rear rank. If this movement be executed in double quick time, each captain, in turn, will halt, and command: *Such company*, *right about*—HALT. At this command, the company designated will face to the right about, and halt.

137. All the companies being aligned, the colonel will cause the guides, who stand faced to the rear, to face about.

Remarks.

138. A column by division at full distance

will close to half distance by the same means and the same commands.

139. A column, by company, or by division, being at full or half distance, the colonel will cause it to close in mass by the same means and commands, substituting the indication, *column, close in mass*, for that of *to half distance, close column.* Each chief of subdivision will conform himself to all that has just been prescribed, except that he will not halt his subdivion till its guide shall be at a distance of six paces from the guide of the subdivision next preceding.

140. In a column, left in front, these various movements will be executed on the same principles.

To march in column at half distance, or close in mass.

141. A column at half distance or in mass, being at a halt, the colonel will put it in march by the commands prescribed for a column at full distance.

142. The means of direction will also be the same for a column at half distance or in

mass, as for a column at full distance, except that the general guides will not step out.

143. In columns at half distance or closed in mass, chiefs of subdivisions will repeat the commands *march* and *halt*, as in columns at full distance.

144. A column by division or company, whether at full or half distance or closed in mass, at a halt or marching, can be faced to the right or left, and marched off in the new direction.

To change direction in column at half distance.

145. A column at half distance, being in march, will change direction by the same commands and according to the same principles as a column at full distance; but as the distance between the subdivisions is less, the pivot man in each subdivision will take steps of fourteen inches instead of nine, and of seventeen inches instead of eleven, according to the gait, in order to clear in time, the wheeling point, and the marching flank will describe the arc of a larger circle, the better to facilitate the movement.

Being in column at half distance, or closed in mass, to take distances.

146. A column at half distance will take full distances *by* the head of the column when it has to prolong itself on the line of battle. If, on the contrary, it has to form itself in line of battle on the ground it occupies, it will take distances *on* the leading or *on* the rearmost subdivision, according as the one or other may find itself at the point where the right or left of the battalion ought to rest in line of battle.

1*st*. *To take distances by the head of the column.*

147. The column being by company at half distance and at a halt, when the colonel shall wish to cause it to take full distances by the head, he will command:

By the head of column, take wheeling distance.

148. At this command, the captain of the leading company will put it in march; to this end, he will command:

1. *First Company, forward.* 2. *Guide left.*
3. MARCH (or *double quick*—MARCH).

149. When the second shall have nearly its wheeling distance, its captain will command:

1. *Second company, forward.* 2. *Guide left.*
3. MARCH (or *double quick*—MARCH).

At the command *march*, which will be pronounced at the instant that this company shall have its wheeling distance, it will step off smartly, taking the step from the preceding company. Each of the other companies will successively execute what has just been prescribed for the second.

150. The colonel will see that each company puts itself in march at the instant it has its distance.

151. If the column, instead of being at a halt, be in march, the colonel will give the same commands, and add:

MARCH (or *double quick*—MARCH).

152. If the column be marching in quick time, at the command *march*, the captain of

the leading company will cause *double quick time* to be taken; which will also be done by the other captains as the companies successively attain their proper wheeling distance.

153. If the column be marching in *double quick time*, the leading company will continue to march at the same gait. The captains of the other companies will cause *quick time* to be taken, and as each company gains its proper distance, its captain will cause it to retake the *double quick step*.

Countermarch of a column at full or half distance.

154. In a column at full or half distance, the countermarch will be executed by the means indicated, School of the Company; to this end, the colonel will command:

1. *Countermarch.* 2. *Battalion right* (or *left*)—FACE. 3. *By file left* (or *right*). 4. MARCH (or *double quick*—MARCH).

To countermarch a column closed in mass.

155. If the column be closed in mass, the countermarch will be executed by the commands and means subjoined.

156. The column being supposed formed by division, right in front, the colonel will command:

1. *Countermarch.* 2. *Battalion, right and left*—FACE. 3. *By file, left and right.* 4. MARCH (or *double quick*—MARCH).

157. At the first command, the chiefs of the odd numbered divisions will caution them to face to the right, and the chiefs of the others to face to the left.

158. At the second command, the odd divisions will face to the right, and the even to the left; the right and left guides of all the divisions will face about; the chiefs of odd divisions will hasten to their right and cause two files to break to the rear, and each chief place himself on the left of the leading front rank man of his division; the chiefs of even divisions will hasten to their left, and cause two files to break to the rear, and each chief place himself on the right of his leading front rank man.

159. At the command *march*, all the divisions, each conducted by its chief, will step off

smartly, the guides standing fast; each odd division will wheel by file to the left around its right guide; each even division will wheel by file to the right around its left guide, each division so directing its march as to arrive behind its opposite guide, and when its head shall be up with this guide, the chief will halt the division, and cause it to face to the front.

160. Each division, on facing to the front, will be aligned by its chief by the right; to this end, the chiefs of the even divisions will move rapidly to the right of their respective divisions.

161. The divisions being aligned, each chief will command, FRONT; at this, the guides will shift to their proper flanks.

162. In a column with the left in front, the countermarch will be executed by the same commands and means; but all the divisions will be aligned by the left; to this end, the chiefs of the odd divisions will hasten to the left of their respective divisions as soon as the latter shall have been faced to the front.

163. In a column by company, closed in mass, the countermarch will be executed by

the same means and commands, applying to company what is prescribed for divisions.

164. The countermarch will always take place from a halt, whether the column be closed in mass, or at full, or half distance.

Being in column by company, closed in mass, to form divisions.

165. The column being closed in mass, right in front, and at a halt, when the colonel shall wish to form divisions, he will command:

1. *Form divisions*. 2. *Left companies, left*—FACE. 3. MARCH (or *double quick*—MARCH).

166. At the first command, the captains of the left companies will caution them to face to the left.

167. At the second command, the left companies will face to the left, and their captains will place themselves by the side of their respective left guides.

168. The right companies, and their captains, will stand fast; but the right and left

guides of each these companies will place themselves respectively before the right and left files of the company, both guides facing to the right, and each resting his right arm gently against the breast of the front rank man of the file, in order to mark the direction.

169. At the command *march*, the left companies only will put themselves in march, their captains standing fast; as each shall see that his company, filing past, has nearly cleared the column, he will command:

1. *Such company.* 2. HALT. 3. FRONT.

170. The first command will be given when the company shall yet have four paces to march; the second at the instant it shall have cleared its right company; and the third immediately after the second.

171. The company having faced to the front, the files, if there be intervals between them, will promptly incline to right; the captain will place himself on the left of the right company of the division, and align himself correctly on the front rank of that company.

172. The left guide will place himself at the same time before one of the three left

files of his company, face to the right, and cover correctly the guides of the right company; the moment his captain sees him established on the direction, he will command:

Right—DRESS.

173. At this, the left company will dress forward on the alignment of the right company; the front rank man, who may find himself opposite to the left guide, will, without preceding his rank, rest lightly his breast against the right arm of this guide; the captain of the left company will direct its alignment on this man, and the alignment being assured, he will command, FRONT; but not quit his position.

174. The colonel seeing the division formed, will command:

Guides—POSTS.

175. At this, the guides who have marked the fronts of divisions will return to their places in column, the left guide of each right company passing through the interval in the centre of the division, and the captains will place themselves as prescribed, No. 75.

176. The colonel, from the directing flank

of the column, will superintend the general execution of the movement.

177. If the column be in march, instead of at a halt, when the colonel shall wish to form divisions, he will command:

1. *Form divisions.* 2. *Left companies, by the left flank.* 3. MARCH (or *double quick*—MARCH).

178. At the first command, the captains of the right companies will command, *Mark time*, the captains of the left companies will caution their companies to *face by the left flank.*

179. At the third command, the right companies will mark time, the left companies will face to the left; the captains of the left companies will each see his company file past him, and when it has cleared the column, will command:

Such company by the right flank—MARCH.

As soon as the divisions are formed, the colonel will command:

4. *Forward.* 5. MARCH.

180. At the fifth command, the column will

resume the gait at which it was marching previous to the commencement of the movement. The guides of each division will remain on the right and left of their respective companies; the left guide of the right company will pass into the line of file closers, before the two companies are united; the right guide of the left company will step into the rear rank. The captains will place themselves as prescribed, No. 75.

Being in column at full or half distance to form divisions.

181. If the column be at a halt, and, instead of being closed in mass, is at full or half distance, divisions will be formed in the same manner; but the captains of the left companies, if the movement be made in quick time, after commanding FRONT, will each place himself before the centre of his company, and command: 1. *Such company, forward.* 2. *Guide right.* 3. MARCH. If the movement be made in double quick time, each will command as soon as his company has cleared the column:

1. *Such company by the right flank.*
2. MARCH.

182. The right guide of each left company will so direct his march as to arrive by the side of the man on the left of the right company. The left company being nearly up with the rear rank of the right company, its captain will halt it, and the movement will be finished as prescribed, No. 371 and following.

183. If the left be in front, the movement will be executed by inverse means; the right companies will conform themselves to what is prescribed above for the left companies; and the two guides, placed respectively, before the right and left files of each left company, will face to the left. At the command, *Guides posts*, given by the colonel, the guides, who have marked the front of divisions, and the captains, will quickly retake their places in the column.

184. If the column be marching at full distance, the divisions will be formed as prescribed, No. 196. If it be marching at half distance, the formation will take place by the

commands and according to the principles indicated, No. 376; if the column be marching in double quick time, the companies which should mark time will march in quick time by the command of their captains.

Remarks on the formation of divisions from a halt.

185. As this movement may be considered as the element of deployments, it ought to be executed with the utmost accuracy.

186. If companies marching by the flank do not preserve exactly their distances, there will be openings between the files at the instant of facing to the front.

187. If captains halt their companies too early, they will want space, and the files which have not cleared the flanks of the standing companies will not be able to dress into line without pushing their ranks laterally.

188. If, on the contrary, the companies be halted too late, it will be necessary for them to incline to the right or left in dressing; and in deployments, either of these faults would lead to error in the following companies.

189. As often as a guide shall have to step out to place himself before his subdivision in order to mark the direction, he will be particularly careful to place himself so as to be opposite to one of the three outer files of the subdivision when they shall be aligned; if he take too much distance, and neither of those files finds itself against him, the chiefs of the subdivision will have no assured point on which to direct the alignment.

1. *Into line, faced to the rear.* 2. *Battalion by the right flank.* 3. MARCH (or *double quick*—MARCH).

190. At the first command, the captains will caution their companies to face by the right flank.

191. At the command *march*, briskly repeated by the captains of companies, all the companies will face to the right; the first company will then wheel by file to the left, and be directed by its captain a little to the rear of the left marker; then pass three paces beyond the line, and wheel again by file to the left; having arrived on the line, the cap-

tain will halt the company, and align it by the right. The remaining part of the movement will be executed as heretofore explained.

192. The foregoing principles are applicable to a column, left in front.

193. As the companies approach the line of battle, it is necessary that their captains should so direct the march as to cross that line a little in rear of their respective guides, who are faced to the basis of the formation; hence each guide ought to detach himself in time to find himself correctly established on the direction, before his company shall come up with him.

Deployment of columns closed into mass.

194. A column in mass may be formed into line of battle:

1. Faced to the front, by the deployment.
2. Faced to the rear, by the countermarch and the deployment.
3. Faced to the right and faced to the left, by a change of direction by the flank, and the deployment.

195. When a column in mass, by division, arrives behind the line on which it is intended to deploy it, the colonel will indicate, in advance, to the lieutenant colonel, the direction of the line of battle, as well as the point on which he may wish to direct the column. The lieutenant colonel will immediately detach himself with two markers, and establish them on that line, the first at the point indicated, the second a little less than the front of division from the first.

196. Deployments will always be made upon lines parallel, and lines perpendicular to the line of battle; consequently, if the head of the column be near the line of battle, the colonel will commence by establishing the direction of the column perpendicularly to line, if it be not already so, by one of the means indicated, No. 244 and following, or No. 307 and following. If the column be in march, he will so direct it that it may arrive exactly behind the markers, perpendicularly to the line of battle, and halt it at three paces from that line.

197. The column, right in front, being halted, it is supposed that the colonel wishes

to deploy it on the first division; he will order the left general guide to go to a point on the line of battle a little beyond that at which the left of the battalion will rest when deployed, and place himself correctly on the prolongation of the markers established before the first division.

198. These dispositions being made, the colonel will command:

1. *On the first division, deploy column.*
2. *Battalion, left* FACE.

199. At the first command, the chief of the first division will caution it to stand fast; the chiefs of the three other divisions will remind them that they will have to face to the left.

200. At the second command, the three last divisions will face to the left; the chief of each division will place himself by the side of its left guide, and the junior captain by the side of the covering sergeant of the left company, who will have stepped into the front rank.

201. At the same command, the lieutenant colonel will place a third marker on the alignment of the two first, opposite to one of the

three left files of the right company, first division, and then place himself on the line of battle a few paces beyond the point at which the left of the second division will rest.

202. The colonel will then command:

3. MARCH (or *double quick*—MARCH).

203. At this command, the chief of the first division will go to its right, and command:

Right—DRESS.

204. At this, the division will dress up against the markers; the chief of the division, and its junior captain, will each align the company on his left, and then command:

FRONT.

205. The three divisions, faced to the left, will put themselves in march; the left guide of the second will direct himself parallelly to the line of battle; the left guides of the third and fourth divisions will march abreast with the guide of the second; the guides of the third and fourth, each preserving the prescribed distance between himself and the

guide of the division which preceded his own in the column.

206. The chief of the second division will not follow its movement; he will see it file by him, and when its right guide shall be abreast with him, he will command:

1. *Second Division.* 2. HALT. 3. FRONT.

207. The first command will be given when the division shall yet have seven or eight paces to march; the second when the right guide shall be abreast with the chief of the division, and the third immediately after the second.

208. At the second command, the division will halt; at the third, it will face to the front, and if there be openings between the files, the chief of the division will cause them to be promptly closed to the right; the left guides of both companies will step upon the line of battle, face to the right, and place themselves on the direction of the markers established before the first division, each guide opposite to one of the three left files of his company.

209. The division having faced to the front

its chief will place himself accurately on the line of battle, on the left of the first division; and when he shall see the guides assured on the direction, he will command, *Right*—DRESS. At this the division will be aligned by the right in the manner indicated for the first.

210. The third and fourth divisions will continue to march; at the command *halt*, given to the second, the chief of the third will halt in his own person, place himself exactly opposite to the guide of the second after this division shall have faced to the front and closed its files; he will see his division file past, and when his right guide shall be abreast with him, he will command:

1. *Third Division.* 2. HALT. 3. FRONT.

211. As soon as the division faces to the front, its chief will place himself two paces before its centre, and command:

1. *Third division, forward.* 2. *Guide right.* 3. MARCH.

212. At the third command, the division will march towards the line of battle; the

right guide will so direct himself as to arrive by the side of the man on the left of the second division, and when the division is at three paces from the line of battle, its chief will halt it and align it by the right.

213. The chief of the fourth division will conform himself (and the chief of the fifth, if there be a fifth) to what has just been prescribed for the third.

214. The deployment ended, the colonel will command:

Guides—Posts.

215. At this command, the guides will resume their places in the line of battle, and the markers will retire.

Remarks on the deployment of columns, closed in mass.

216. All the divisions ought to deploy rectangularly, to march off abreast, and to preserve their distances towards the line of battle.

217. Each division, the instant that it is unmasked, ought to be marched towards the line of battle, and to be aligned upon it by the flank

next to the directing division; the latter, whether the right or left be in front, will always be aligned by the flank next to the point of *appui*, when the deployment is made on the first or last division; but if the column be deployed on an interior division, this division will be aligned by the flank which *was* that of direction.

218. The chiefs of division will see that, in deploying, the principles prescribed for marching by the flank are well observed, and if openings between the files occur, which ought not to happen, except on broken or difficult grounds, the openings ought to be promptly closed towards the directing flank as soon as the divisions face to the front.

219. If a chief of division give the command *halt*, or the command, *by the right* or *left flank*, too soon or too late, his division will be obliged to oblique to the right or left in approaching the line of battle, and his fault may lead the following sub-division into error.

220. In the divisions which deploy by the left flank, it is always the left guide of each company who ought to place himself on the

line of battle, to mark the direction; in divisions which deploy by the right flank, it is the right guide.

221. A column by company, closed in mass, may be formed to the left or to the right into line, in the same manner as a column at half distance, and by the means indicated, No. 502, and following.

222. A column by company, closed in mass, may be formed on the right or on the left into line of battle, as a column at half distance; but in order to execute this movement, without arresting the march of the column, it is necessary that the guides avoid, with the greatest care, shortening the step in turning, and that the men near them, respectively, conform themselves rapidly to the movements of their guides.

To march by the flank.

223. The colonel, wishing the battalion to march by the flank, will command:

1. *Battalion.* 2. *Right* (or *left*)—FACE. 3. *Forward.* 4. MARCH (or *double quick*—MARCH).

224. At the second command, the captains

and covering sergeants will place themselves as prescribed, Nos. 136 and 141, School of the Company.

225. The sergeant on the left of the battalion will place himself to the left and by the side of the last file of his company, covering the captains in file.

226. The battalion having to face by the left flank, the captains, at the second command, will shift rapidly to the left of their companies, and each place himself by the side of the covering sergeant of the company preceding his own, except the captain of the left company, who will place himself by the side of the sergeant on the left of the battalion. The covering sergeant of the right company will place himself by the right side of the front rank man of the rearmost file of his company, covering the captain in file.

227. At the command *march*, the battalion will step off with life; the sergeant, placed before the leading file (right or left in front), will be careful to preserve exactly the length and cadence of the step, and to direct himself straight forward; to this end, he will take points on the ground.

228. Whether the battalion march by the right or left flank, the lieutenant colonel will place himself abreast with the leading file, and the major abreast with the color-file, both on the side of the front rank, and about six paces from it.

229. The adjutant, placed between the lieutenant-colonel and the front rank, will march in the same step with the head of the battalion, and the sergeant major, placed between the major and the color-bearer, will march in the same step with the adjutant.

230. The captain and file closers will carefully see that the files neither open out, nor close too much, and that they regain insensibly their distances, if lost.

231. The colonel wishing the battalion to wheel by file, will command:

1. *By file right* (or *left*). 2. MARCH.

232. The files will wheel in succession, and all at the place where the first had wheeled, in conforming to the principles prescribed in the School of the Company.

233. The battalion marching by the flank, when the colonel shall wish it to halt, he will command:

1. *Battalion*. 2. HALT. 3. FRONT.

234. These commands will be executed as prescribed in the School of the Company, No. 146.

235. If the battalion be marching by the flank, and the colonel should wish to cause it to march in line, either to the front or to the rear, the movements will be executed by the commands and means prescribed in the School of the Company.

Changes of front.

Change of front perpendicularly forward.

236. The battalion being in line of battle, it is supposed to be the wish of the colonel to cause a change of front forward on the right company, and that the angle formed by the old and new positions be a right angle, or a few degrees more or less than one; he will cause two markers to be placed on the new direction, before the position to be occupied by that company, and order its captain to establish it against the markers.

237. The captain of the right company will

immediately direct it upon the markers by a wheel to the right on a fixed pivot; and after having halted it, he will align it by the right.

238. These dispositions being made, the colonel will command:

1. *Change front forward on first company.* 2. *By company, right half wheel.* 3. MARCH (or *double quick*—MARCH).

239. At the second command, each captain will place himself before the centre of his company.

240. At the third, each company will wheel to the right on the fixed pivot; the left guide of each will place himself on its left as soon as he shall be able to pass; and when the colonel shall judge that the companies have sufficiently wheeled, he will command:

4. *Forward.* 5. MARCH. 6. *Guide right.*

241. At the fifth command, the companies ceasing to wheel will march straight forward; at the sixth, the men will touch elbows towards the right.

242. The right guide of the second company will march straight forward until this company shall arrive at the point where it should turn to the right; each succeeding right guide will follow the file immediately before him at the cessation of the wheel, and will march in the trace of this file until this company shall turn to the right to move upon the line; this guide will then march straight forward.

243. The second company having arrived opposite to the left file of the first, its captain will cause it to turn to the right; the right guide will direct himself so as to arrive squarely upon the line of battle, and when he shall be at three paces from that line, the captain will command:

1. *Second company.* 2. HALT.

244. At the second command, the company will halt; the files not yet in line with the guide will come into it promptly, the left guide will place himself on the line of battle, and as soon as he is assured in the direction by the lieutenant-colonel, the captain will align the company by the right.

245. Each following company will conform to what has just been prescribed for the second.

246. The formation ended, the colonel will command:

Guides—Posts.

247. If the battalion be in march, and the colonel shall wish to change front forward on the first company, and that the angle formed by the old and new positions be a right angle, he will cause two markers to be placed on the new direction, before the position to be occupied by that company, and will command:

1. *Change front forward on first company.* 2. *By company, right half wheel.* 3. March (or *double quick*—March).

248. At the first command, the captains will move rapidly before the centre of their respective companies; the captain of the first company will command: 1. *Right turn;* 2. *Quick time;* the captains of the other companies will caution them to wheel to the right.

249. At the command *march*, the first company will turn to the right according to the prin-

ciples prescribed in the School of the Soldier, No. 402; its captain will halt it at three paces from the markers, and the files in rear will promptly come into line. The captain will align the company by the right.

250. Each of the other companies will wheel to the right on a fixed pivot; the left guides will place themselves on the left of their respective companies, and when the colonel shall judge they have wheeled sufficiently, he will command:

4. *Forward.* 5. MARCH. 6. *Guide right.*

251. These commands will be executed as indicated No. 746 and following.

252. The colonel will cause the battalion to change front forward on the eighth company according to the same principles and by inverse means.

Remarks on changes of front.

253. When the new direction is perpendicular, or nearly so, to that of the battalion, the companies ought to make about a *half wheel* (the eighth of the circle) before marching, straight forward; but when those two

lines are oblique to each other, the smaller the angle which they form, the less ought the companies to wheel. It is for the colonel to judge, according to the angle, the precise time when he ought to give the command *march*, after the caution *forward*, and if he cannot catch the exact moment, the word of execution should rather be given a little too soon than an instant too late.

Dispositions against cavalry.

254. A battalion being in column by company at full distance, right in front, and at a halt, when the colonel shall wish to form it into square, he will first cause divisions to be formed; which being done, he will command:

1. *To form square.* 2. *To half distance, close column.* 3. MARCH (or *double quick* —MARCH.

255. At the command *march*, the column will close to company distance, the second division taking its distance from the rear rank of the first division.

256. At the moment of halting the fourth division, the file closers of each company of

which it is composed, passing by the outer flank of the companies, will place themselves two paces before the front rank opposite to their respective places in line of battle, and face towards the head of the column.

257. At the commencement of the movement, the major will place himself on the right of the column abreast with the first division; the buglers formed in two ranks will place themselves at platoon distance, behind the inner platoons of the second division.

258. These dispositions being made, the colonel may, according to circumstances, put the column to march or cause it to form square; if he wish to do the latter, he will command:

1. *Form square.* 2. *Right and left into line, wheel.*

259. At the first command, the lieutenant colonel, facing to the left guides, and the major, facing to those of the right, will align them, from the front, on the respective guides of the fourth division, who will stand fast, holding up their pieces, inverted, perpendicularly; the right guides, in placing themselves on the direction, will take their exact distances.

260. At the second command, the chief of the first division will caution it to stand fast; all the captains of the second and third divisions will place themselves before the centres of their respective companies, and caution them that they will have to wheel, the right companies to the right, and the left companies to the left into line of battle.

261. The chief of the fourth division will command: 1. *Fourth division, forward;* 2. *Guide left*, and place himself at the same time two paces outside of its left flank.

262. These dispositions ended, the colonel will command:

MARCH (or *double quick*—MARCH).

263. At this command, briskly repeated, the first division will stand fast; but its right file will face to the right, and its left file to the left.

264. The companies of the second and third divisions will wheel to the right and left into line, and the buglers will advance a space equal to the front of a company.

265. The fourth division will close up to form the square, and when it shall have closed, its

chief will halt it, face it about, and align it by the rear rank upon the guides of the division, who will, for this purpose, remain faced to the front. The junior captain will pass into the rear rank, now become the front, and the covering sergeant of the left company will place himself behind him in the front rank, become rear. The file closers will, at the same time close up a pace on the front rank, and the outer file on each flank of the division will face outwards.

266. The square being formed, the colonel will command:

Guides—Posts.

267. At this command, the chiefs of the first and fourth divisions, as well as the guides will enter the square.

268. The captains whose companies have formed to the right into line, will remain on the left of their companies; the left guide of each of those companies, will, in the rear rank, cover his captain, and the covering sergeant of each will place himself as a file closer behind the right file of his company.

269. The fronts of the square will be designated as follows; the first division will always

be the *first front;* the last division, the *fourth front;* the right companies of the other divisions will form the *second front;* and the left companies of the same divisions the *third front.*

270. A battalion being in column by company, at full distance, right in front, and in march, when the colonel shall wish to form square, he will cause this movemement to be executed by the commands and means indicated, No. 817.

271. At the command *march*, the column will close to company distance, as is prescribed, No. 278. When the chief of the fourth division shall command *Quick, march*, the file closers of this division will place themselves before the front rank.

272. If the colonel shall wish to form square he will command:

1. *Form square.* 2. *Right and left into line, wheel.* 3. MARCH.

273. At the first command, the chief of the first division will caution it to halt; all the captains of the second and third divisions will rapidly place themselves before the centres of their respective companies, and caution them that they will have to wheel, the right companies to

the right, and the left companies to the left into line. The chief of the fourth division will caution it to continue its march, and will hasten to its left flank. At the third command, briskly repeated, the chief of the first division will halt his division and align it to the left, the outer files will face to the right and left, the rest of the movement will be executed as prescribed No. 828 and following.

274. The first and fourth fronts will be commanded by the chiefs of the first and fourth divisions; each of the other two by its senior captain.

275. The commander of each front will place himself four paces behind its present rear rank, and will be replaced momentarily in the command of his company by the next in rank therein.

276. The battalion being formed into square, when the colonel shall wish to cause it to advance a distance less than thirty paces, he will command:

1. *By* (such) *front, forward.* 2. MARCH.

277. If it be supposed that the advance be made by the first front, the chief of this front will command:

1. *First division, forward.* 2. *Guide centre.*

278. The chief of the second front will face his front to the left. The captains of the companies composing this front will place themselves outside, and on the right of their left guides, who will replace them in the front rank; the chief of the third front will face his front to the right, and the captains in this front will place themselves outside, and on the left of their covering sergeants; the chief of the fourth front will face his front about, and command:

1. *Fourth division, forward.* 2. *Guide centre.*

The captain, who is in the centre of the first front, will be charged with the direction of the march, and will regulate himself by the means indicated in the School of the Company, No. 89.

279. At the command *march*, the square will put itself in motion; the companies marching by the flank will be careful not to lose their distances. The chief of the fourth division will cause his division to keep constantly closed on the flanks of the second and third fronts.

280. If the colonel should wish to halt the square, he will command:

1. *Battalion.* 2. HALT.

281. At the second command, the square will halt; the fourth front will face about immediately, and without further command; the second and third fronts will face outwards; the captains of companies will resume their places as in square.

282. In moving the square forward by the second, third, or fourth fronts, the same rule will be observed.

283. The battalion being formed into square, when the colonel shall wish to cause it to advance a greater distance than thirty paces, he will command:

1. *Form column.*

284. The chief of the first division will command:

1. *First division, forward.* 2. *Guide left.*

285. The commander of the fourth front will caution it to stand fast; the commander of the second front will cause it to face to the left, and then command, *By company, by file left.* The commander of the third front will cause it to face to the right, and then command:

By company, by file right. At the moment the second and third fronts face to the left and right, each captain will cause to break to the rear the two leading files of his company.

To reduce the square.

286. The colonel, wishing to break the square, will command:

1. *Reduce square.* 2. MARCH (or *double quick*—MARCH).

287. This movement will be executed in the manner indicated, No. 863 and following; but the file closers of the fourth front will place themselves behind the rear rank the moment it faces about; the field and staff, the color-bearer and buglers, will, at the same time, return to their places in column.

Squares in four ranks.

288. If the square formed in two ranks, according to the preceding rules, should not be deemed sufficiently strong, the colonel may cause the square to be formed in four ranks.

289. The battalion being in column by company at full distance, right in front, and at a halt, when the colonel shall wish to form

square in four ranks, he will first cause divisions to be formed, which being executed, he will command:

1. *To form square in four ranks.* 2. *To half distance, close column.* 3. MARCH (or *double quick*—MARCH).

290. At the first command, the chief of the first division will caution the right company to face to the left, and the left company to face to the right. The chiefs of the other divisions will caution their divisions to move forward.

291. At the command *march*, the right company of the first division will form into four ranks on its left file, and the left company into four ranks on its right file. The formation ended, the chief of this division will align it by the left.

292. The other divisions will move forward and double their files marching; the right company of each division will double on its left file, and the left company on its right file. The formation completed, each chief of division will command, *Guide left.* Each chief will halt his division when it shall have the distance of a company front in four ranks

from the preceding one, counting from its rear rank, and will align his division by the left. At the instant the fourth division is halted, the file closers will move rapidly before its front rank.

293. The colonel will form square, re-form column, and reduce square in four ranks by the same commands and means as prescribed for a battalion in two ranks.

294. If the square formed in four ranks be reduced and at a halt, and the colonel shall wish to form the battalion into two ranks, he will command :

1. *In two ranks undouble files.* 2. *Battalion outwards*—FACE. 3. MARCH.

295. At the first command, the captains will step before the centres of their respective companies, and those on the right will caution them to face to the right, and those on the left, to face to the left.

296. At the second command, the battalion will face to the right and left.

297. At the command *march*, each company will undouble its files and re-form into two ranks as indicated in the School of the

Company, No. 376 and following. Each captain will halt his company and face it to the front. The formation completed, each chief of division will align his division by the left.

Remarks on the formations of squares.

298. It is a general principle that a column by company, which is to be formed into square, will first form divisions, and close to half distance. Nevertheless, if it find itself suddenly threatened by cavalry, without sufficient time to form divisions, the colonel will cause the column to close to platoon distance and then form square by the commands and means which have been indicated; the leading and rearmost companies will conform themselves to what has been prescribed for division in those positions. The other companies will form by platoon to the right and left into line of battle, and each chief of platoon, after having halted it, will place himself on the line, as if the platoon were a company, and he will be covered by the guide in the rear rank.

299. A battalion in column at full distance having to form a square, will always close on the leading subdivision; and a column closed

in mass, will always, for the same purpose, take distances by the head. In either case, the second subdivision should be careful, in taking its distance, to reckon from the rear rank of the subdivision in front of it.

300. If a column by company should be required to form square in four ranks, the doubling of files will always take place on the file next the guide.

301. When a column, disposed to form square, shall be in march, it will change direction as a column at half distance; thus having to execute this movement, the column will take the guide on the side opposite to that to which the change of direction is to be made, if *that* be not already the side of the guide.

302. A column doubled on the centre at company distance or closed in mass, may be formed into square according to the same principles as a simple column.

303. When a battalion is ployed, with a view to the square, it will always be in rear of the right or left division, in order that it may be able to commence firing, pending the execution of the movement. The double column, also, affords this advantage, and be-

ing more promptly formed than any other, it will habitually be employed, unless particular circumstances cause a different formation to be preferred.

304. A battalion, in square, will never use any other than the fire by file and by rank; the color being in the line of file closers, its guard will not fall back as prescribed No. 41; it will fire like the men of the company of which it forms a part.

305. If the square be formed in four ranks, the first two ranks will alone execute the firings prescribed above; the other two ranks will remain either at shoulder or support arms.

306. The formation of the square being often necessary in war, and being the most complicated of the manœuvres, it will be as frequently repeated as the supposed necessity may require, in order to render its mechanism familiar to both officers and men.

307. In the execution of this manœuvre, the colonel will carefully observe that the divers movements which it involves succeed each other without loss of time, but also without confusion; for, if the rapidity of cavalry movement requires the greatest prompti-

tude in the formation of squares, so, on the other hand, precipitancy always results in disorder, and in no circumstance is disorder more to be avoided.

THE END.

www.ingramcontent.com/pod-product-compliance
Lightning Source LLC
Chambersburg PA
CBHW030405270326
41926CB00009B/1276